Kamado Smoker And Grill Cookbook

*The Ultimate Kamado Smoker and Grill Cookbook –
Innovative Recipes and Foolproof Techniques for The Most
Flavorful and Delicious Barbecue'*

Table of Contents

Introduction

Thank you for purchasing this book, '*Kamado Smoker and Grill Cookbook - The Ultimate Kamado Smoker and Grill Cookbook – Innovative Recipes and Foolproof Techniques for The Most Flavorful and Delicious Barbecue.*'

Have you been ordering meals from outside quite often? Are you bored of home-cooked food? Are you spending a significant amount of your paycheck on food? If you have answered yes to any of these three questions, the chances are that you need to find out what's keeping you from eating home food. Using the same cooking techniques and the same old boring recipes can make you want to eat our restaurants all the time. After all, who likes to eat the same kind of food every day? Are you someone like me who loves a bit of smoky flavor in her meats? How about some home-cooked barbecued food with a bit of rustic flavor to it? Sounds perfect, isn't it?

If you have used barbecue grills before and you found them to be too messy to use, the Kamado smoker and grill is your best bet. This magical ceramic cooker can add the much-needed flavor and taste to your otherwise bland dishes. We all love the smell of some delicious food cooked over some burning charcoals. Food cooked in the Kamado is not only flavorful but also moist and delectable. With the Kamado, you can have a barbecue party almost every weekend without spending too much time or energy.

This book offers you all the information you ever wanted to know about the Kamado smoker and grill. We have explained every bit about the Kamado smoker and grill in detail to make it easier for beginners to learn how to handle it. This guide includes vital information like types of Kamado grills, how to operate it, tips for managing the device and a conversion chart.

Besides educating our readers about this device, we also wanted to present you with some lip-smacking recipes that easy to follow and can be prepared in no time. We know how difficult it can get to experiment with your food amidst this busy life. In today's times, where we are struggling to spend time with our loved ones, spending some more on cooking can seem imaginable. We all want to come home to some sumptuous food after a long day at work. When you start using the Kamado grill and smoker, you will never want to order food from a restaurant. We assure you that buying this well-engineered and remarkable equipment will be worth every penny you spend. Happy reading!!

Chapter 1: What is a Kamado Smoker and Grill?

If you are a fan of smoked meats, I am sure you know what a Kamado is. For the rest of you who don't, it's just another name for a grill. The name "Kamado" means the stove in Japanese. One of the most popular versions of the Kamado grill is known as "The Big Green Egg." Have you ever spotted a big green pot at the shopping mall, which looks a little bit like a stove? That's a Kamado. This traditional Japanese earthen vessel has become increasingly popular in the American market for its reliability, ease of use and versatility. You can make a variety of delectable dishes using the Kamado and relish on them while enjoying the company of your loved ones.

The Kamado grill is inarguably one of the best units that are capable of holding extremely high and low temperatures at the same time, making them perfect for smoking and grilling. There are about ten different types of Kamado grills, which are priced between $500 USD and $4000 USD and are available in various sizes and colors.

- Big Green Egg – Large: One of the most popular models, this Kamado grill can cook up a 20-pound turkey at one go.
- Saffire Kamado Bronze class Grill and Smoker
- Primo Oval XL Charcoal Grill
- Komodo Kamado OTB 23-inch Charcoal Grill
- Vision Grills Kamado Grill
- Broil King Keg Charcoal Grill
- Kamado Joe Classic
- Black Olive Pellet Kamado Grill
- Grill Dome Infinity Series – large
- Char-Broil Kamander

What makes a Kamado different?

The Kamado is earthenware that can perform several functions at the same time such as grilling, braising, barbecuing and searing. This is the only barbecuing device that comes with a dual wall construction like a thermos bottle. The firebox inside the grill has walls that are about 6 inches thick, whereas the walls at the grill levels are almost 4 inches thick. This high insulating quality helps in cooking the food within no time and with a minimal amount of lump wood charcoal. Other grills are made of metal and require a lot of coals to make up for the lost heat. When you use more coals, you also need a lot of air flows to keep the temperatures consistent. This air can also quickly dry out the meats and cause them to shrink. The Kamado, on the other hand, doesn't need a lot of charcoal. Owing to its extreme efficiency, you require fewer briquettes, which are completely burned while cooking. This results in a lot of moisture retention and the meats turn out to be more juicer and tender.

How to light the Kamado?

- Start by removing the grill gently and crumbly about 3 or 4 sheets of paper (newspaper). Now place them straight on top of the grate.
- Next, place two or three (6inch) pieces of kindling wood over the paper.
- Put enough number of briquettes over the newspaper and the wood.
- Light the newspaper using a matchstick and let it burn for about 40 to 60 seconds before you close the dome.
- Now close the lid. Take off the damper top and gently open the slide draft door. Keep it wide open.
- Start waving a piece of cardboard or a magazine paper to start the draft. Keep waving it right on the front side of the draft door so the air can be forced into the Kamado. Now you can stop fanning, as the Kamado will keep naturally drawing the air.
- You can see that within the first 5 minutes of the kindling and the paper burning away, the charcoal will start to light. Now quickly start spreading the fire using a poker, so the charcoal starts burning brightly. Now, wait for another 5 minutes, so the charcoal to get red-hot.
- Place the grill back and allow it to warm up for about 2-3 minutes before you start adding the meat.

- The briquettes won't take more than 15 minutes to get ready. This means you can utilize this time to assemble your ingredients.
- Start adjusting the heat by restricting the airflow through the draft door as well as the damper.
- If you wish to refuel the Kamado, simply add about 1 to 6+ briquettes by lifting the grill slightly and slipping in the charcoal via the slots on the ring.

How to control the temperatures?

The key to nailing a perfect dish in the Kamado is to monitor the temperatures. You may need a little effort, in the beginning, to understand about the temperature controls, but once you get the hang of it, it will become easier. You can achieve the perfect temperature through draft control by adjusting the top for the damper as well as the draft door. If you love gorging on smoky flavored meats, you can simply close damper top and leave the draft door open. When you leave the draft door open 2/3 and the damper top open 1/3, it will give you the same temperature results as the draft door 1/3 and the damper top 2/3. If you find this method slightly confusing at the start, you can also use a thermometer for checking the temperature of the Kamado.

Chapter 2: History of Kamado Grills

The legacy of Kamado grills goes back about thousands of years. The Kamado is based on ancient-technology and the earliest cooking vessels found in China dated over 3,000 years old. Even though several clay Kamado were found in the ruins of early civilizations, it's difficult to guess its exact origin. It has also found its roots in India, which was carbon dated to more than 4000 years ago. Let's look at how the Kamado has evolved from merely being a clay pot used to cook food to this remarkably efficient and snazzy looking device.

Ancient Cooking in Ceramics

Since the beginning of time, our ancestors often used clay pots to cook food. These cookers were used by almost everyone, as clay was readily available. Every household would have at least one large clay pot, in which they would cook their family meals. Several archaeologists have found these cooking pots made of clay in almost every part of the world. The interesting thing to note is that some of these clay pots have a striking resemblance to the Kamado grills & smoker. Cooking in these clay pots always enhanced the flavors and added a mouth-watering taste to the dishes. Ceramic clay pots still have the same magic associated with cooking.

The Mushikamado (Rice Cooker)

People from different parts of the world cooked their staple foods in the ceramic pots. But they all had different styles of cooking, and the pots too differed in shape and size. The Japanese used a remarkably different device that was used for cooking rice. This device looked very distinct from the other pots and the rice cooked in it tasted better too. This rice cooker was called the "MushiKamado," and was used to cook rice for family dinners and ceremonial occasions. However, one could not barbecue or grill meat or anything else in this rice cooker.

The MushiKamado, a Japanese invention, was made completely out of clay, and it looked pretty much like most cooking vessels around the globe. The same rice cooker, also known as the MushiKamado, is widely known as the Kamado grills today and is getting increasingly popular across the globe. The MushiKamado was a circular pot with a domed lid that could be lifted off the base. It also came with a draft door as well as a damper. The MushiKamado had a rice pot inside it, which was suspended on top of the "fire box" using a fire ring. Charcoal was used as a source of fuel to generate heat and food could be cooked on very high as well as extremely low temperatures.

How did the MushiKamado become the Kamado?

In the 1960's, a man named Richard Kamado redesigned and patented the MushiKamado rice cooker and turned it into a ceramic barbecue pot. Mr. Johnson named his new barbecue grill, the Kamado, a word that had no descriptive meaning. Soon the newly designed Kamado was trade marked by him and became a necessary device, which was used for multiple purposes. Unlike, the older version of the Kamado, one could use this grill not only for cooking rice but also for smoking grilling and barbecuing meats and other foods. Richard opened a Kamado factory in the southern part of Japan and upgraded the grill with a sliding draft door, hinged bands, grill and other significant improvements.

More than a thousand Kamados were sold for as low as $12 to the U.S Air force crew, who would bring these Kamados back in unoccupied military transport planes. Initially, they found it difficult to ship the fragile Kamado pots, but soon Richard invented the crate, and the shipping process was simplified. Later, over 1,00,000 Japanese Kamados were shipped by them. The Kamados were marketed perfectly well in the U.S market, with every major departmental store displaying them. These stores included Bullocks, Rich's in Atlanta, Neiman Marcus, Macy's, Breuners and J.W. Robinsons. Furthermore, the Kamados was also featured in popular magazines such as playboy, sunset, and Esquire. These Kamados were so long-lasting that a lot of the early purchasers still use them for cooking. Richard Johnson had claimed that the Kamado grill is "the barbecue grill in the world," and many people would still agree with this.

The American Kamado

Richard Johnson, later in the 1960's manufactured some ceramic Kamado grills in the United States. These Kamados were made from high fire ceramics and used a high gloss ceramic glaze. These Kamados rectified two of primary problems associated with the

Japanese Kamado: One that would no longer crack with heat and the second one was that the glaze worked as a better option to retain the color.

Today's Kamado

The Kamado Company, in the year 1996, introduced a brand new ceramic tiled Kamado. This product was not only better looking, but it cooked better too. Richard Johnson, the patent holder of the Kamado, had researched and developed this new device in California. Today, the Kamado is far more aesthetically pleasing and serves as a life-long functional product that can be used to cook some delicious food in no time.

Chapter 3: Kamado Grill and Smoker Basics

How does a Kamado work?

Working with the Kamado is incredibly simple. While cooking, the air flows straight through the bottom, over the coals and then travels out on top. The coals get hotter as they get more air, but if devoid of oxygen, can take a long time to cool down. The best way to use a Kamado is to manage the amount of airflow. There are two vents attached to the Kamado, one at the bottom and the other at the top. As you get done with cooking, you need to close both the vents completely. This helps in cutting off the oxygen supply to the coals, and the fire goes kaput.

When you first get a Kamado home, you need to buy some good quality lump charcoal, which will act as a fuel. The next step is to cook some yummy pork-butt. This pork needs to be slowly cooked and burn in the Kamado for about 24 hours. This process is called curing and is done to prolong the shelf life of the Kamado pot. But that doesn't mean that you can't cook anything else while the pot is going through this process. You can simply cook some pork roast on the grill while the curing process is on. But you need to ensure that the temperature is not more than 200 degrees.

Lighting the grill

To start with, open the bottom vent properly and then the damper to have the maximum airflow. Gather your lump charcoal and pile it up on either side of the grill basin. You can't cook all the recipes using direct heat. Piling colas on a single side of the grill can help you to place the food on the other side, thereby avoiding direct heat. Now you don't need to fill the grill basin completely with charcoal. You can use about a shoe box size of lump charcoal, which will be enough for cooking about 6 quarts of food. However, if you are going to cook longer, you are certainly going to require more charcoal.

Reaching the desired temperature

The first and foremost thing you need to do is to get the coals way hotter than needed, and then cool them down. For instance, if you are going to slow cook some lamb legs at 200 degrees, let your Kamado heat up to 300 degrees. Later, get the top and bottom vents closed completely so the temperature drops. To get the Kamado down to 200 degrees, only slight air is required to trickle through. The type of charcoal you are using determines how closed or open your vents should be. Hence, it's important to stick to your favorite brand of lump wood charcoal as it saves you a lot of guesswork regarding you don't have to figure out how to adjust the air flow inside the pot.

You may not know this, but the bottom vent adjusts the temperatures by about 10 degrees with the slightest of adjustment. On the other hand, the damper on top adjusts the temperatures by 5 degrees with each turn. The take away from this information is that adjusting the bottom vent can be key to reach your desired temperate, making your cooking easier.

Cooking

I can't instruct you a lot here. Everyone has his or her way of cooking in the Kamado. The biggest advantage of using a Kamado grill and smoker is its temperature control, so make optimum use of it to cook your dishes. Besides that, the kiln-like atmosphere inside the pot helps in keeping the food moist for longer periods. It also avoids unwanted flare up and keeps the food from burning. Remember not to open the lid frequently while the food is cooking away. Each time you open the lid of the pot, a little flavor gets chipped away. Keep the vents closed unless you need to add additional ingredients to the dish.

Safety

The Kamado grill and smoker is practically safe for use. There's nothing much that you need to know about its safety beyond your common sense. That being said, here's an important tip - Be sure to open your Kamado lids carefully, especially when the food is hot. Remember that cooking in Kamado requires a lot of oxygen starvation. So, when you open the lid in a hurry, the hot coals might just flare up right on your face. WHOOOSH! Who wants an accidental burn! I bet no one wants to risk causing burn wounds. But if you always carefully open the lid of the pot, you will face absolutely no issue.

Cleaning

This one may seem redundant, but the cleaning of the Kamado grill and smoker is extremely vital for its life span. While the cleaning part may seem overwhelming to you, the good news is that if you use high-quality lump wood charcoal along with the efficient burns does not leave you with a lot of ash, unlike the other grills. You will be relieved to know how infrequently you are required to remove the ashes simply by using good quality charcoal. On the slightly negative side, the pile of ash can restrict the airflow, so as much as you would like to avoid cleaning it often, you will have to do it anyway.

Now, for getting out the ash through the bottom vent, will require a little patience. You will have to remove the ash through the basin, compelling you to carry out the dirty job of taking out the left over coals. This process may sound a bit overwhelming, but it's not too bad if you follow our tips mentioned below.

The damper

The damper acts like a giant screw and needs to be cleaned now and then. Keeping the damper clean will prevent it from getting it stuck and increase its lifespan. So, clean the damper at least once or twice every month by unscrewing it completely and washing it with a bit of soapy water. Try lubricating the damper before you put it back.

The outer parts of the Kamado

Since the modern Kamado is made of ceramic tiles, you can use an all-purpose kitchen cleaner to keep it shiny and spotless. You can also use some soap-water and a napkin to clean the Kamado covering.

The inside of the cooking chamber

We all wish that the cream-colored insides of the Kamado stay just the same, but it doesn't work that way. Don't get too freaked out by the little grime that starts building up once you start using the Kamado. Every once a while, clean the insides of the grill gate. After you are done cooking the food, don't just close off the grill. Instead, allow the vents to remain open and let the temperature get up to 600 degrees. Let it the pot burn with the lid still on until the coals completely vanish. Following this exact process may not be necessary, but it will certainly make your life easier.

Final tip

The clay air sieve, which is at the bottom of the Kamado, has about a dozen holes for allowing the air to pass through it. Now, these holes may invariably get clogged with ash or tiny pieces of lump charcoal. What you can do is fit in a small wire grill grate that permits more air to flow upwards, and more ash to flow downwards. This helps in keeping the temperatures consistent and makes them easier to control.

Chapter 4: Reasons for buying a Kamado Grill and Smoker - Pros and Cons

Primary reasons to buy the Kamado grill and smoker.

Ease of use

Besides being reliable and sturdy, it's also a very easy appliance to use. Numerous factors make this unit extremely user-friendly. Some of them are mentioned below:

- Assembly time for this unit usually doesn't amount to more than 20-30 minutes. This means you can start grilling on the same day of purchase and have a delicious meal within no time.
- Most Kamado models come with a user-friendly thermometer that can save you a lot of guesswork for calculating the time taken for the grill to heat up. It can also help you in gauging the exact time as to how long our food may need to get cooked.
- Start-up time for the grill is typically around 15 minutes, thereby, allowing you enough time to gather your ingredients without spending a lot of time waiting for it to perfect the temperature.
- The Kamado grill needs minimal maintenance. All you need to do is perform an annual test to check the tightness of band screws and gaskets. Always remember to change the gaskets once every 2 or three years to maintain optimal performance of your grill.
- You can easily clean the grill by simply using a brush or scrape the cooking grate.
- The Kamado grills are typically around 18.5 inches, leaving you a lot of space to move around in the kitchen. They can be pushed inside a grill table for creating additional space and are perfect for outdoor locations.

Efficiency and versatility

The fact that Ceramic Kamado grills often work on lump wood charcoal separates them from the rest of the competition. Using lump wood charcoal for grilling produces less ash as compared to the other grills in the market. This makes it even easier to clean and sustainable. The material used for constructing the Kamado grills along with its creative design makes it retain more heat as compared to other products. The heat is distributed evenly throughout the grill, and you can set the temperatures as high as 750+ F or as low as 225 F. Also, the Kamado grill is capable of holding the low temperatures uniformly for over 12 hours, making it ideal for smoking meats.

Besides grilling and smoking, the Kamado grill can also be used for baking some bread or even pizza. This grill operates the same way as the wood-fired ovens. You can use them to bake just about anything that you may consider baking in a traditional oven. Few of the top-end Kamado grill models are capable of handling a rotisserie cradle, which is considered to be a great way of browning the meats. Regardless of whether you wish to smoke, grill, bake or roast, Kamado grills may just be the perfect appliance you have been searching for.

One grill, three different cooking styles

Direct Cooking

Direct cooking involves placing the food straight on to the grill grate, right over the heat source. This commonly used technique is largely effective in cooking ingredients that require lesser cook time. These ingredients may include tender veggies or thin-cut chops. Direct cooking results in faster cook time, typically taking about not more 6 minutes to complete.

Indirect Cooking

Indirect cooking on Kamado utilizes an internal heat barrier that is capable of efficiently diffusing the heat from the charcoal. The heat deflector inside the Kamado is either curved or circular based on the design of your grill. This deflector aims at maintaining the airflow for regulating the temperature inside the grill. Indirect cooking creates a charcoal fired oven like environment that can handle temperatures ranging from 200 F to 650F.

Raised direct cooking

For direct cooking, you can cook the food directly over the coals by placing it about three inches away from the fire, which results in fast cook time. For raised cooking, on the other hand, the food is placed about 8 to 10 inches away from the fire for preventing it from violent delivery of heat. This allows the food to cook slower while enhancing the flavors of the dish. Through raised cooking, the food benefits from the heat that radiates from the dome. This type of cooking style also ensures that your food is slowly brought to a particular temperate for achieving the desired levels of doneness. Raised cooking is a wonderful way to make crispier and crunchier consistency in food.

Smoking (Slow and low cooking)

The Kamado smoker works perfectly well with low and slow cooking temperatures. The food is typically smoked at 225 F over a period of 5 to 15 hours. You can also add wood chips by placing them around the charcoal for smoldering while the food is cooking away. Animal parts such as ribs, shoulders or muscles that are harder and slower to cook can benefit the most from slow and low cooking. During the slow cooking process, the connective tissues, as well as the collagens, start melting away, leaving behind the juicy and tender meat. Traditionally, slow and low cooking forms the basis of barbecue cooking and brings out the best flavors of the food.

Advantages of Kamado grill and smoker

Quality

Even though the higher versions of the Kamado grills may seem slightly expensive, they are made of fine quality materials. The ceramic outer coating ensures that your pot retains the color and looks relatively new even after years of usage. You know some of the people who have been using the Kamado for the longest time suggest that you don't pick a Kamado in color you like, instead you get one in which your kids like, as it will be passed on to them when you die. I think that says a lot about its durability too.

Taste

Cooking in ceramic grill and smoker offers tastier food as compared to the food cooked in gas or briquette charcoal grills. Since the Kamado uses lump charcoal, which is made from hardwoods such as maple, oak, and hickory, it can bring out the optimum flavors of the food.

Moisture retention

Owing to its innovative shape, it offers excellent heat circulation and insulation. The food can be cooked at extremely low temperatures as well. It requires very little heat to cook, which results in many moist dishes. Whereas the other grills lack temperature control, resulting in moisture loss.

Year-around usage
You can use the Kamado about 12 months of the year regardless of the season. Since the food is cooked in a closed pot, it is not subjected to the weather conditions.

Less Startup time
The Kamado grill and smoker takes just about 15 minutes for the assembly. This saves you from having to wait too long for the unit to heat up and reduces your cooking time.

Temperature range
The Kamado grill and smoker is perfectly capable of maintaining consistent temperatures as high as 750 F and as low as 225 F easily. Besides that, you can also retain the low temperature for over 12 hours for smoking.

Heat source
The Kamado grill uses natural lump charcoal as a source of fuel, making it inexpensive for usage. Most professional and competitive chefs prefer using natural lump charcoal for cooking food, as it is 100% natural. This type of fuel can burn hotter, cleaner and longer as compared to other sources of fuel.

Fuel cost
Since the natural lump charcoal is quite inexpensive, you won't have to worry too much about the fuel costs. While the price of natural lump charcoal is comparatively lower, ensure that you don't end up buying a ridiculously cheaper charcoal, which is produced using a lot of chemicals and additives. If it's way too cheap, then it's not natural lump charcoal. Six quarts of natural lump charcoal can be used for a single cooking session and can cost you around $1.50-$1.75 depending on where you buy it from and the brand.

Cleaning and maintenance
Kamado grills produce about one-third of that ash produced by briquettes. You can easily brush or scrape the grate before you start cooking. Briquette needs a lot of brushing due to the amount of ash it produces, whereas the natural gas needs about 15 minutes or so to clean the grates. Overall, the Kamado grills are comparatively easier to maintain.

Kamado Grill and Smoker cons

You may not want to hear one bad word about your favorite device. But like all other devices, there's always room for improvement with regards to the Kamado too. Although we are sure that the positives aspects of using the Kamado are enough to override its negatives, it's important that you know everything about the device you are buying. So here are a few downsides to using this new age device.

Two-zone grilling is difficult
The inability to perform zonal grilling is probably going to disappoint you a bit at the beginning when you first buy the product. For those of you who don't know what two zone grilling is, it's when the grill is split up in two areas at a different temperature. So, grilling a dish at a high temperature on one side and the other at low temperature on the other side seems a little difficult. However, with the new Kamado grilling accessories in the market, such as the grill expanders and the heat deflectors, two-zone cooking might just be achievable.

Fragile
Yes, ceramics are brittle, and the weight of the dome could mean if it drops, it's likely to crack a little bit. But once you get the hang of this slightly fragile device, handling it wouldn't be such a problem. After all, Kamados are pretty long-lasting pots that can stay with you for years to come.

Heavy
They may be fragile, but the Kamado grills are certainly not lightweight. If you are thinking about a 162/172 kg for their best selling model, it can be a struggle for an average person to lift it. But hey, we can always use a wheel-cart for helping us with the ease of movement. Just keep in mind that it's a ceramic grill, and you may need some help to move it from one end to the other carefully.

Outer dome can get hot
This is not a great point to bash this gentle device, but we don't want you to stay uninformed. Since Kamado grills are capable of cooking food as high as 750F, the lid of the pot is obviously going to get the hottest at a high temperature like that. Now we are not saying that it can get scalding hot such as traditional BBQ, but you need to use a hand towel to open the lid. But if you are a patient person, you may just wait for a few minutes and let the lid cool off a bit before trying to open it.

Chapter 5: Kamado Grilling Recipes

Tokyo Teriyaki Chicken

Ingredients:

- 2-3 pounds chicken breast halves, with skin, rinsed, pat dried
- 1 teaspoon fresh ginger, peeled, grated
- 1 teaspoon Coahuila sauce
- ½ teaspoon salt or to taste
- ½ cup soy sauce
- 2 cloves garlic, peeled, crushed
- 3 tablespoons white wine or sherry

Method:

1. Operate the grill following the instructions of the manufacturer. Set the Kamado grill for grilling with the temperature at 350 ° F for about 25-30 minutes.
2. Place lava stone and heat deflector bracket.
3. Add soy sauce, garlic, ginger, wine, Coahuila sauce and salt into a big bowl.
4. Add chicken and coat it well with the mixture. Let it marinate in the mixture for at least 2 hours.
5. Place the chicken with its skin side down on the surface of the lower grill. Grill the chicken for 4-6 minutes. Flip sides and grill the other side for 4-6 minutes or until a meat thermometer when inserted in the thickest portion of the meat shows 175-180 ° F.
6. Remove the chicken from the grill and cover loosely with foil for 10 minutes.
7. Serve.

Bacon Wrapped Chicken Kabobs

Ingredients:

- 2 packages chicken tenders, cut into 1-inch pieces
- BBQ seasoning as required
- 2 packages thin-sliced bacon
- BBQ sauce as required

Method:

1. Operate the grill following the instructions of the manufacturer. Set the Kamado grill for grilling with the temperature at 400 ° F for about 25-30 minutes.
2. Place a drip pan on the bottom shelf and a diffuser.
3. Wrap the bacon around the chicken and insert the skewer into the wrapped bacon. Repeat with the remaining bacon slices and chicken pieces. You may need 2-3 skewers to fit all the bacon wrapped chicken pieces into it.
4. Sprinkle BBQ rub on the bacon wrapped chicken pieces.
5. Place the skewers on the topmost rack of the grill. Let it cook for 15-20 minutes. Turn the skewers around. As the chicken cooks, in a while, the bacon will begin to have brown spots on it. Cook for another 5-6 minutes or until done.
6. Remove from the skewers. Brush BBQ sauce over it.
7. Serve with extra BBQ sauce if desired.

Grilled Garlic Lemon Chicken

Ingredients:

- 6 chicken breasts
- Juice of 3 lemons
- A handful fresh parsley, chopped
- 4 teaspoons garlic, minced
- Salt to taste
- Pepper powder to taste
- 6 tablespoons extra virgin olive oil
- Few thin slices lemon

Method:

1. Add olive oil, salt, pepper, garlic, parsley and lemon juice into a zip lock bag.
2. Add chicken and shake the bag so that the chicken is well coated with the marinade. Place in the refrigerator for 1 hour.
3. Operate the grill following the instructions of the manufacturer. Set the Kamado grill for grilling with the temperature at 400 ° F for about 25-30 minutes.
4. Place chicken directly on the grill. Place lemon slices on the chicken. Close the dome and cook until the chicken is tender or until a meat thermometer when inserted in the thickest portion of the meat shows 160 ° F. Let the chicken rest for 5 minutes.
5. Sprinkle remaining parsley and serve.

Plank Grilled Chicken with Fruit Salsa

Ingredients:

- 1 ½ cups fresh peach, chopped
- ¾ cup red bell pepper, chopped
- 1 ½ cups fresh mango, peeled, pitted, chopped into small pieces
- 1/3 cup onion, thinly sliced
- 4 tablespoons lime juice + extra to serve
- Salt to taste
- 6 chicken breasts (6 ounces each), skinless, boneless
- Lime wedges to serve
- 1/3 cup fresh basil leaves, torn
- 3 teaspoons olive oil
- 1 alder plank, soaked for an hour

Method:

1. Add peach, mango, onion, bell pepper, and lime juice into a bowl. Mix well. Cover and set aside for a while for the flavors to set in.
2. Operate the grill following the instructions of the manufacturer. Set the Kamado grill for grilling with the temperature at 325 ° F for about 25-30 minutes.
3. Brush chicken with olive oil. Rub it well. Sprinkle salt.
4. Place plank on the grid close to the dome. Let it heat for a minute. Turn the plank and place chicken on the heated side.
5. Grill for 20 minutes or until a meat thermometer when inserted in the thickest portion of the meat shows 165-174 ° F.
6. When done, drizzle lime juice over the grilled chicken.
7. Add basil into salsa. Stir and serve with grilled chicken.

Creole Shrimp with Grilled Rice

Ingredients:

- 1 ½ pounds Andouille sausage
- 2 pounds large shrimp, peeled
- 2 cans (16 ounces each) Cajun or regular stewed, chopped tomatoes
- 2 bell peppers, chopped
- 6 cloves garlic, finely chopped
- ½ cup fresh cilantro, chopped
- 2 medium onions, chopped
- 2 stalks celery, chopped
- 1 cup green onions, chopped
- 2 bay leaves
- 2 cups white wine
- 2 cups water
- 8 tablespoons butter, divided
- ½ cup flour
- Salt to taste
- Pepper to taste
- 4 cups short grain white rice
- Creole seasoning to taste
- Louisiana hot sauce to serve (optional)

Method:

1. To make Creole sauce: Place a pan over medium heat. Add half the butter. When butter melts, add flour and constantly stir for a couple of minutes until fragrant.
2. Add onion, garlic, celery and bell pepper and sauté for 8-10 minutes.
3. Stir in the tomatoes, water, bay leaf, white wine, cilantro, Creole seasoning and green onions.
4. Lower heat. Cover and simmer for about 45 minutes. Stir frequently. The final sauce should be thin in consistency. Discard the bay leaf. Cover and set-aside until use.

5. Cook rice according to the instructions on the package. The cooked rice should be sticky. Cool the cooked rice for about 10 minutes.

6. Divide the rice into 6-8 portions and shape into patties. Brush top of the patties with butter.

7. Thread shrimp and sausage on separate skewers.

8. Operate the grill following the instructions of the manufacturer. Set the Kamado grill for grilling with the temperature at 400 ° F for about 25-30 minutes.

9. Place a drip pan on the bottom shelf and a diffuser.

10. Place the rice patties on the grill with the butter side facing down on the coolest part of the grill. Grill for 5 minutes. Brush the top of patties with butter. Flip sides and grill the other side for 4-5 minutes. Remove the patties.

11. Place skewers with sausages on the grill. Grill for 3 minutes. Turn the skewer and now place the skewers with shrimp. Cook for 2 minutes and turn the skewers with shrimp. Cook for 2 minutes or until pink.

12. To serve: Place a patty on each serving plate. Pour Creole sauce over the patty. Serve with shrimp and sausages.

Reverse Seared Porterhouse Steak

Ingredients:

- 2 porterhouse steaks (1.75 inches thick each), at room temperature
- Salt to taste or steak seasoning to taste
- Pepper powder to taste
- 2 tablespoons butter, melted

Method:

1. Operate the grill following the instructions of the manufacturer. Set the Kamado grill for grilling with the temperature at 250 ° F for about 25-30 minutes. Use the heat deflector.
2. Brush all the butter over the steaks. Sprinkle steak seasoning or salt and pepper over it.
3. Place steaks directly on the grill. Cook until a meat thermometer when inserted in the thickest portion of the meat shows 115 ° F.
4. When done, wrap the steak tightly in foil. Remove the heat deflector.
5. Raise the temperature to around 650 ° F and open up the vents of the Kamado grill.
6. Sear for half a minute on each side leaving the dome open while searing. A meat thermometer when inserted in the thickest portion of the meat shows 130 ° F for medium rare.
7. Remove from the grill and let it rest for 10 minutes before serving.

Grilled Pork Chops

Ingredients:

<u>For pork:</u>

- 16 cups basic brine
- 8 Porterhouse pork chops

<u>For the rub:</u>

- 2 tablespoons smoked paprika
- 4 teaspoons salt
- 1 teaspoon granulated garlic
- ½ teaspoon cayenne pepper
- 4 teaspoons sugar
- 4 teaspoons light brown sugar
- 1 teaspoon pepper powder

<u>For the glaze:</u>

- 4 tablespoons sorghum syrup
- 3 teaspoons soy sauce
- 2/3 cup red pepper jelly
- 2 tablespoons butter, unsalted

Method:

1. Add brine into a large container. Add pork chops into it. Place in the refrigerator for 2-4 hours.
2. Meanwhile, add all the ingredients for the glaze into a saucepan. Place the saucepan over medium low heat. Heat the mixture until well combined. Remove from heat. Cover and set aside.

3. Operate the grill following the instructions of the manufacturer. Set the Kamado grill for grilling with divided cooking, with the temperature at 350 ° F for about 25-30 minutes.
4. Remove the pork chops from the refrigerator. Remove from brine and pat the chops dry. Sprinkle the rub over it. Rub it in lightly.
5. Lay the pork chops on the higher grill to ensure indirect cooking.
6. Grill for 20-30 minutes or until a meat thermometer when inserted in the thickest portion of the meat shows 120-130 ° F. Remove the chops from the higher grill and set aside for a while.
7. Raise the temperature to above 500 ° F by increasing the ventilation.
8. Place the chops on the lower grid. Sear for 2 minutes on each side.
9. Pour glaze on top and serve.

Grilled Meatballs

Ingredients:

- 3 pounds ground beef
- 1 ½ tablespoons dried basil
- 1 ½ cups panko bread crumbs
- 1 ½ tablespoons granulated garlic
- 3 teaspoons dried oregano
- 1 ½ teaspoons pepper powder
- 1 ½ teaspoons salt
- 3 eggs
- 1/3 cup Romano cheese or parmesan cheese, grated

Method:

1. Add all the ingredients into a bowl. Mix well with your hands until well combined.
2. Shape into balls of about 2 inches diameter. Place on a pan that is greased with oil. Cover the pan with foil tightly.
3. Operate the grill following the instructions of the manufacturer. Set the Kamado grill for grilling with the temperature at 400 ° F with plate setter with legs down.
4. Place a pizza stone on top of the plate setter. Place the pan on it in the middle, along with the foil.
5. Let it cook for 25 minutes. Discard the foil and cook for another 10 minutes or until the meatballs are brown.
6. Remove the pan from the grill and let it cool for 5 minutes. Place the meatballs on a plate that is lined with paper towel.
7. Serve over spaghetti with a sauce of your choice. You can also insert toothpicks in the meatballs and serve as an appetizer.

Steak and Shrimp Fajitas

Ingredients:

For fajitas:

- 2 pounds skirt steak
- 2 large onions, peeled, sliced
- 12-15 large portabella mushrooms, sliced along with the stems
- 2 limes
- 1-pound large shrimp, peeled, deveined
- 4 bell peppers of different colors, sliced thinly
- 4 jalapeño peppers, thinly sliced
- Olive oil or vegetable oil

For marinade:

- Juice of 2 limes
- 4 cloves garlic, finely chopped, smashed
- 2 teaspoons ground cumin
- 4 tablespoons Worcestershire sauce
- ½ cup tequila or wine vinegar or red wine
- 2 tablespoons fresh cilantro, chopped
- 1 teaspoon ground cayenne pepper
- 2 teaspoons pepper powder or to taste

Toppings: Use as required

- Salsa
- Cheese, shredded
- Flour tortillas
- Lettuce leaves, chopped
- Guacamole

Method:

1. To make marinade: Add all the ingredients of the marinade into a bowl and whisk well. Add skirt steaks and mix well. Transfer into a zip lock bag. Seal the bag and refrigerate for 8-24 hours.
2. Remove from the refrigerator an hour before grilling. Discard the marinade and rinse lightly. Pat the steaks dry and brush with oil.
3. Operate the grill following the instructions of the manufacturer. Set the Kamado grill for raised grilling with the temperature at 425 ° F for about 15-20 minutes.
4. Place a cast iron skillet or fajita skillet on the grill. Brush oil on the bottom of the skillet.
5. When the skillet is heated, add all the fajita ingredients except shrimp. Grill until tender. It should take 10-15 minutes.
6. Top the grilled vegetables with shrimp and cook for 3-5 minutes. Place the skirt steaks on the grill. Grill for a minute. Flip sides and grill the other side for a minute. Remove the steaks and set aside on your cutting board.
7. When the shrimp are cooked, remove the pan from the grill.
8. When the steaks are cool enough to handle, slice steak along the grain.
9. Warm the tortillas according to the instructions on the package.
10. Serve steaks and grilled vegetables with shrimp along with the toppings.

Sizzling Diablo Shrimp

Ingredients:

- 1 cup butter
- 2 teaspoons cayenne pepper
- 1 cup white wine
- 2-3 pounds shrimp, peeled, deveined, with tail
- Freshly ground pink peppercorns
- 8 cloves garlic, minced
- 2 teaspoons ground cumin
- ½ cup flat leaf parsley, chopped
- 1 teaspoon coarse salt

Method:

1. Operate the grill following the instructions of the manufacturer. Set the Kamado grill for grilling with the temperature at 350 ° F. Place lava stone or pizza stone. Let it preheat for 20 minutes.
2. Meanwhile, place a saucepan over medium low heat. Add butter. When butter melts, add garlic, cayenne pepper and cumin and sauté until garlic is soft.
3. Add wine. Scrape the bottom of the saucepan to remove any browned bits that are stuck.
4. Increase the heat to high and boil until the liquid in the saucepan is reduced to half its original quantity. Remove from heat and cool for a while.
5. Add parsley and stir.
6. Place shrimp in a bowl. Pour the wine mixture over it. Season with salt and toss until well coated.
7. Transfer the shrimp on to the lava stone. Grill for 3-4 minutes. Flip sides half way through grilling.
8. Serve hot.

Bacon Wrapped Tenderloins

Ingredients:

- 4 pork tenderloins, trimmed of fat, discard silver skin
- 3 tablespoons green peppercorns packed in water, drained
- 15-16 fresh, large sage leaves
- 1 teaspoon freshly ground sea salt
- 6 tablespoons Dijon style mustard
- 6 tablespoons coarsely grounded 5 peppercorns blend (which is made by mixing equal parts of black pepper, green pepper, white pepper, pink pepper and whole allspice and grinding it coarsely)
- 18-20 slices bacon
- Few 10-inch bamboo skewers or metal skewers (soak in water for 30 minutes if using bamboo skewers or brush olive oil on the metal skewers)

Method:

1. Operate the grill following the instructions of the manufacturer. Set the Kamado grill for grilling with the temperature at 350 ° F. Place lava stone or pizza stone on top of the cooking grate. Let it preheat for 20 minutes.
2. Sprinkle salt over the tenderloins.
3. Make a cut lengthwise with a sharp knife along the center of the tenderloin up to 2/3 the thickness.
4. Open up the meat and flatten it slightly. Brush mustard all over the tenderloin. Sprinkle green pepper corns all over the opened meat and press the peppercorns lightly using your hands.
5. Sprinkle about 2 tablespoons of the 5 peppercorns blend all over the opened meat. Lay the sage leaves along the center of the meat.
6. Close the tenderloin back to its original shape.
7. Take the bacon slices and wrap it all around the tenderloins. Fasten by inserting the skewers through bacon wrapped tenderloins.
8. Place the skewers with tenderloins on the grill on the hottest part. Grill for about 10 minutes. Turn the tenderloins. It should be brown on all the sides.
9. Now shift the tenderloins to the upper grill. Grill for 20-30 minutes or until a meat thermometer when inserted in the thickest portion of the meat shows 145 ° F. Remove the chops from the higher grill and cover loosely with foil. Set aside for a while.
10. Slice the tenderloins diagonally and serve.

Grilled Sweet Potato Wedges

Ingredients:

- 8 medium sweet potatoes, scrubbed, cut into 8 equal wedges each
- 2 tablespoons fresh parsley leaves, chopped to garnish
- ½ cup olive oil

For seasoning:

- 2 teaspoons paprika
- 2 teaspoons chili powder
- Salt to taste
- Freshly ground black pepper to taste
- 2 teaspoons ground cumin
- ¼ teaspoon cayenne pepper

Method:

1. Operate the grill following the instructions of the manufacturer. Set the Kamado grill for grilling with the temperature at 350 ° F. Place the cooking grate in its position and cover the grill. Let it preheat for 5 minutes. Grease the grilling grate.
2. To make seasoning: Add all the ingredients of seasoning into a bowl and mix well. Set aside.
3. Add potato wedges to a bowl. Drizzle oil over it. Toss until well coated. Sprinkle salt and pepper over it.
4. Place the sweet potatoes on the cooler part of the grill. Cook until tender. It can take 30-40 minutes. Push the sweet potatoes to the hottest part of the grill and cook for 2 minutes on each side until it is brown all over.
5. Remove the sweet potatoes from the grill and place on a serving platter. Sprinkle seasoning over it. Garnish with parsley and serve right away.

Eggplant Caprese

Ingredients:

- 2 large eggplants, cut into ¼ inches slices, crosswise
- 4 large tomatoes, cut into ¼ inch thick slices
- 2 tablespoons kosher salt
- 1-2 tablespoons balsamic vinegar
- 2 large balls fresh mozzarella, cut into ¼ inch thick slices
- ½ cup basil chiffonade
- Extra virgin olive oil, as required
- Freshly ground pepper to taste

Method:

1. Place a colander in a large bowl. Place eggplant slices in the colander. Sprinkle salt over the slices and toss well. Some moisture will be drained into the bowl.
2. After about 30 minutes, pat the eggplant slices dry with paper towels.
3. Operate the grill following the instructions of the manufacturer. Set the Kamado grill for grilling with the temperature at 350 ° F. Place the cooking grate in its position and cover the grill. Let it preheat for 5 minutes. Grease the grilling grate.
4. Brush oil on both sides of the eggplant. Place it directly on the grill and cook until brown on both the sides. It should take around 4-5 minutes.
5. Place a slice of eggplant on a serving plate. Layer with a slice of tomato followed by a slice of mozzarella. Place another slice of eggplant over it followed by tomato and mozzarella. Finally, place a slice of eggplant on top. Drizzle oil and vinegar. Sprinkle pepper and basil. Serve right away.
6. Repeat the above step with the remaining ingredients.

Grilled Cabbage with Blue Cheese Dressing

Ingredients:

- 2 medium head cabbages, cut into 6 wedges each (do not remove the core)
- ½ cup scallions
- 1 cup bacon, cooked, crumbled (optional)
- 8 ounces blue cheese, crumbled, mashed
- 1 cup sour cream
- Kosher salt to taste
- Freshly ground pepper to taste
- 4 tablespoons extra virgin olive oil
- 2 cups cherry tomatoes, half if desired
- 1 cup mayonnaise
- 2 tablespoons lemon juice
-

Method:

1. Add blue cheese, mayonnaise, salt, pepper, lemon juice and sour cream into a bowl. Whisk until well combined. Set aside.
2. Operate the grill following the instructions of the manufacturer. Set the Kamado grill for grilling with the temperature at 350 ° F. Place the cooking grate in its position and cover the grill. Let it preheat for 5 minutes. Grease the grilling grate.
3. Place cabbage directly on the hottest part of the grill and cover the dome. Cook until charred on all the 3 sides. It should take around 4-5 minutes.
4. Push the cabbage to the cooler side of the grill. Cover and cook for 3-4 minutes or until crisp as well as tender in the center.
5. Transfer to a bowl. Drizzle oil. Toss well. Sprinkle salt and pepper and toss again.
6. Drizzle blue cheese sauce over it. Top with scallions, tomatoes, and bacon and serve.

Grilled Kale Salad with Warm Bacon Vinaigrette

Ingredients:

- 2 pounds Tuscan or dinosaur kale, discard hard stems and ribs
- Kosher salt to taste
- Freshly ground pepper to taste
- 2 small shallots, minced
- 6 tablespoons extra virgin olive oil, divided
- 6 slices bacon, chopped
- ½ cup apple cider vinegar

Method:

1. Operate the grill following the instructions of the manufacturer. Set the Kamado grill for grilling with the temperature at 350 ° F. Place the cooking grate in its position and cover the grill. Let it preheat for 5 minutes. Grease the grilling grate.
2. Add kale into a large bowl. Drizzle 4 tablespoons oil and toss. Sprinkle salt and pepper and toss well.
3. Place kale on the grill. Cover and grill for a couple of minutes until slightly charred.
4. Flip sides and cover again. Grill until slightly charred.
5. Meanwhile, place a heavy bottomed skillet over medium heat. Add remaining oil. When the oil is heated, add bacon and sauté for a minute. Add shallots and stir.
6. Cook until the bacon is crisp. Add vinegar and simmer until thick.
7. Remove the kale from the grill and chop it. Pour dressing on top. Toss well.
8. Serve immediately.

Grilled Fruit Cobbler

Ingredients:

- 7-8 cups berries or fruit of your choice
- 2 tablespoons cornstarch
- 2 tablespoons milk
- ½ cup sugar
- 3-4 cans refrigerated biscuits

Method:

1. Operate the grill following the instructions of the manufacturer. Set the Kamado grill for grilling with the temperature at 350 ° F. for 10 minutes.
2. Take a cast iron skillet. Add fruit, cornstarch, and 6 tablespoons sugar. Mix until well combined.
3. Place the refrigerated biscuits over the fruit layer. Brush the biscuits with milk.
4. Sprinkle 2 tablespoons sugar.
5. Place the skillet on the grill. Close the dome and cook for 15 minutes or until the biscuits are light brown. Check the color of the biscuits after 7-8 minutes every 2-3 minutes. It should not brown too much.

Banana Butter Pecan Kabobs

Ingredients:

- 21 ounces frozen pound cake, thawed, cubed
- ½ cup butter, melted
- 1 teaspoon vanilla extract
- 1 cup butterscotch ice cream topping
- 4 large bananas, peeled, cut into 1 inch thick slices
- 4 tablespoons brown sugar
- ¼ teaspoon ground cinnamon
- 1 cup pecans, chopped, toasted
- 8 cups butter pecan ice cream to serve

Method:

1. Take 7-8 metal skewers or wooden skewers (if using wooden skewers, then soak in water for 30 minutes). Thread cake cubes and banana slices alternately on to the skewers.
2. Mix together in a bowl, butter, vanilla, brown sugar, and cinnamon. Brush this mixture over the banana and cake pieces.
3. Place the skewers on the topmost rack of the grill. Close the dome of the grill. Let it cook for 4-5 minutes or until brown. Turn the skewers around after 2 minutes of grilling. Grill in batches if required.
4. Serve warm in bowls. Scoop some ice cream into the bowls. Trickle some butterscotch topping. Garnish with pecans and serve.

Chapter 6: Kamado Smoking Recipes

Baby Back Ribs

Ingredients:

- 4 pounds pork loin ribs, trimmed, discard membrane from back of each rack
- 1 teaspoon ground celery seeds
- 2 tablespoons onion salt
- 4 tablespoons paprika
- 4 teaspoons hot sauce
- 1 teaspoon cayenne pepper
- 1/3 - ½ cup garlic salt
- 2 teaspoons sage
- 2 cups apple juice

Method:

1. Add all the dry ingredients into a bowl and mix well.
2. Sprinkle this mixture on the pork loin on both the sides. Rub it into the pork. Place in the refrigerator for a minimum of 2 hours.
3. Operate the grill following the instructions of the manufacturer. Set the temperature between 175-200° F for about 25-30 minutes.
4. Place a rib rack, lava stone, and heat deflector bracket.
5. Place 3-6 wood chunks of your choice or 3-5 handfuls chips over the charcoal for smoking. Close the dome until you place the meat.
6. Lay the ribs on the grill. Close the dome. Cook for 5-6 hours. Baste with apple juice every 50-60 minutes until done.

Smoked Pork Roast

Ingredients:

- 4-6 pounds pork roast
- BBQ rub of your choice, as required

Method:

1. Sprinkle rub on the pork roast on both the sides. Rub it into the pork. Place at room temperature until the grill heats.
2. Operate the grill following the instructions of the manufacturer. Set the temperature between 225-250° F for about 25-30 minutes.
3. Place 3-6 wood chunks of your choice or 3-5 handfuls chips over the charcoal for smoking. Close the dome until you place the meat.
4. Place the roast on the grill. Close the dome. Cook for 5-6 hours or until done.

Smoked Spareribs

Ingredients:

- 3 racks spareribs, peeled

For the rub:

- 6 tablespoons paprika
- 6 tablespoons granulated garlic
- 3 tablespoons raw sugar
- 6 tablespoons sugar
- 3 tablespoons pepper powder
- 3 tablespoons dried oregano
- 6 tablespoons kosher salt
- 3 tablespoons chili powder
- 3 tablespoons onion powder
- 3 tablespoons dried thyme

For BBQ sauce:

- ¾ cup sugar
- ¾ teaspoon dried thyme
- 3 teaspoons kosher salt
- ¾ cup white vinegar
- 1 ½ cups tomato ketchup
- 2 teaspoons cayenne pepper
- 1 ½ teaspoons dried oregano
- 1 ½ teaspoons pepper powder
- 1 ½ cups molasses
- 1 ¼ cups yellow mustard
- 1 ½ teaspoons granulated garlic

Method:

1. To make the rub: Add all the ingredients of rub into a bowl. Mix well. Rub the mixture all over the spareribs. Place the spareribs on a large sheet of foil and wrap it. Place in the refrigerator for 7-8 hours.
2. Remove the spareribs an hour before smoking.
3. Operate the grill following the instructions of the manufacturer. Set the temperature between 245° F for about 25-30 minutes.
4. Place 3-6 cherry wood chunks or wood chunks of your choice or 3-5 handfuls chips over the charcoal for smoking. Close the dome until you place the meat.
5. Place the spareribs on the grill. Close the dome. Cook for 3 – 3 ½ hours.
6. Remove the spareribs from the grill and wrap in foil. Place the wrapped spare ribs and cook for 2-3 hours. Remove from the grill and let it sit for an hour.
7. Meanwhile, make the BBQ sauce as follows: Add all the ingredients of the sauce into a saucepan. Place the saucepan over medium heat. Simmer until well combined.
8. Pour BBQ sauce over the spareribs and serve.

Smoked Brisket

Ingredients:

- 4 pounds brisket
- 1-2 tablespoons yellow mustard
- 1-2 tablespoons Worcestershire sauce

For the rub:

- ½ tablespoon kosher salt
- 1 tablespoon brown sugar
- ½ teaspoon cayenne pepper
- ½ teaspoon minced, dried onions
- 1 tablespoon black pepper powder
- 1 tablespoon chili powder
- ½ teaspoon ground cumin
- 1 tablespoon red pepper flakes
- 1 tablespoon paprika

For Mop ingredients:

- ½ can beer
- ½ teaspoon kosher salt
- 2 cloves garlic, minced
- ½ cup apple cider vinegar
- ½ tablespoon brown sugar
- ½ tablespoon red pepper flakes

Method:

1. Add all the rub ingredients into a bowl and mix well.
2. Rub yellow mustard and Worcestershire sauce on the cold brisket.
3. Sprinkle dry mixture on the brisket. Place at room temperature for a while.
4. Operate the grill following the instructions of the manufacturer. Set the temperature between 225-250° F for about 25-30 minutes.

5. Place a drip pan on the bottom shelf.
6. Place 3-6 oak wood chunks or wood chunks of your choice or 3-5 handfuls chips over the charcoal for smoking. Close the dome until you place the meat.
7. Mix together all the ingredients of a mop in a bowl.
8. Place meat on the grill. Close the dome. Cook for 5-6 hours. Brush with a mop after an hour of cooking. After that, brush mop every 40-45 minutes until meat thermometer when inserted in the thickest portion of the meat shows 190 ° F. Remove the chops from the higher grill and cover with 2 layers of heavy duty foil.
9. Cover with a towel. Set aside for 1 – 1-½ hours.
10. Serve.

Smoked Beef Back Ribs

Ingredients:

- 2-3 beef ribs, trimmed
- Beef rub of your choice, as required
- Yellow mustard, as required

Method:

1. Remove the ribs from the refrigerator an hour before smoking.
2. Operate the grill following the instructions of the manufacturer. Set the Kamado grill for indirect grilling with the temperature at 225 ° F for about 25-30 minutes.
3. Spread mustard liberally all over the ribs. Sprinkle rub all over the ribs.
4. Place 3-6 pecan wood chunks or wood chunks of your choice or 3-5 handfuls chips over the charcoal for smoking. Close the dome until you place the meat.
5. Place meat on the grill. Close the dome. After 2 hours of cooking, rotate the grill grate by 180 °. Squirt some apple juice over it if desired and cook for 2-3 hours. Check every 30 minutes so that the meat is not burnt. Squirt some more juice if required until done. Cook until done.

Smoked Meatloaf

Ingredients:

- 4 pounds ground beef
- 4 stalks celery, finely chopped
- 6 cloves garlic, minced
- 4 tablespoons Worcestershire sauce
- 2 teaspoons red wine vinegar
- 2 tablespoons fresh rosemary, minced
- 4 teaspoons salt or to taste
- 2 cups onion, finely chopped
- 2 carrots, grated
- 4 cups panko bread crumbs
- 1 cup red wine
- 6 eggs
- 2 tablespoons fresh thyme, minced
- ½ tablespoon paprika
- 1 cup ketchup
- 2 teaspoons olive oil

Method:

1. Operate the grill following the instructions of the manufacturer. Set the Kamado grill for smoking with the temperature at 350 ° F. Place the cooking grate in its position and cover the grill. Let it preheat for 10 minutes.
2. Meanwhile, place a pan over medium heat. Add oil. When the oil is heated, add onion, celery, and carrots and cook until onions are translucent.
3. Add garlic and sauté until fragrant. Remove from heat.
4. Attach the paddle attachment to a mixer. Add sautéed vegetables and mix until well combined. Add an egg at a time and mix well each time.
5. Add fresh herbs, wine, breadcrumbs, vinegar, and spices. Mix well.
6. Grease a loaf pan with butter and transfer the meat mixture into it.

7. Place 3-6 apple wood chunks or wood chunks of your choice or 3-5 handfuls chips over the charcoal for smoking. Close the dome until you place the meat.
8. Place loaf pan on the grill. Close the dome. Cook for 20-30 minutes. Remove the loaf pan from the grill and brush ketchup liberally on the top.
9. Smoke for another 10-12 minutes. Add more wood chunks if necessary.
10. Cook until meat thermometer when inserted in the center of the loaf shows 155 ° F.

Smoking Chicken

Ingredients:

- 6-8 pieces chicken, rinsed, pat dried
- 1 tablespoon salt or to taste
- Freshly ground pepper to taste
- 2 tablespoons packed brown sugar
- 2 tablespoon Sriracha sauce

Method:

1. Operate the grill following the instructions of the manufacturer. Set the Kamado grill for smoking with the temperature at 225-250 ° F for about 25-30 minutes.
2. Add sugar, salt, and pepper into a bowl. Spread this mixture on the chicken. Place the chicken in a large re-sealable bag. Place in the refrigerator for 2-6 hours.
3. Place 3-6 mesquite or hickory wood chunks or wood chunks of your choice or 3-5 handfuls chips over the charcoal for smoking. Close the dome until you place the meat.
4. Place chicken with skin side down on the grill. Cook for 1 ½ - 2 hours or until meat thermometer when inserted in the thickest portion of the meat shows 170-175 ° F. Remember that leg and thigh pieces take longer than the breast pieces to cook.

Greek Chicken

Ingredients:

- 1 whole chicken of about 3-4 pounds
- 2 tablespoons Greek seasoning
- Pepper to taste
- Seasoning salt to taste
- BBQ sauce, as required (optional)

Method:

1. Operate the grill following the instructions of the manufacturer. Set the Kamado grill for smoking with the temperature at 225 ° F for about 25-30 minutes.
2. Sprinkle seasoning, salt, and pepper on the chicken. Rub it well on to the chicken.
3. Place 3-6 mesquite or hickory wood chunks or wood chunks of your choice or 3-5 handfuls chips over the charcoal for smoking. Close the dome until you place the meat.
4. Place chicken with skin side down on the grill. Cook for 1 ½ - 2 hours or until meat thermometer when inserted in the thickest portion of the meat shows 160-165 ° F.
5. If you are using BBQ sauce, then spread it on the chicken during the last 10 minutes of cooking.
6. Serve hot.

Lemon Pepper Chicken

Ingredients:

- 1 whole chicken of 3-4 pounds
- 2 lemons, chopped into 8 pieces each
- ¼ cup lemon juice
- Freshly ground pepper to taste
- Salt to taste

Method:

1. Sprinkle some lemon juice over the chicken. Place the lemon pieces into the cavity of the chicken.
2. Sprinkle pepper generously over the chicken. Also, sprinkle salt over it. Refrigerate for 1-2 hours.
3. Operate the grill following the instructions of the manufacturer. Set the Kamado grill for smoking with the temperature at 300 ° F for about 25-30 minutes.
4. Place 3-6 mesquite or hickory wood chunks or wood chunks of your choice or 3-5 handfuls chips over the charcoal for smoking. Close the dome until you place the meat.
5. Place chicken with skin side down on the grill. Cook for 1-1 ½ hours or until meat thermometer when inserted in the thickest portion of the meat shows 160-165 ° F. Rotate the chicken

Smoked Turkey

Ingredients:

- 10 -15 pounds turkey
- 2 tablespoons vegetable oil
- ½ tablespoon pepper powder
- 10 cloves garlic, chopped
- 1 apple, cored, quartered
- 1 medium onion, chopped
- 3-4 tablespoons soy sauce

For brine:

- 1 cup kosher salt
- ½ bottle white wine
- ½ bottle red wine
- 1 cup chicken broth
- 2-3 navel oranges
- 2 large onions, chopped coarsely
- 4 bay leaves
- 2 tablespoons whole peppercorns
- 2 tablespoons whole cloves
- 1 medium head garlic, peeled, chopped
- 2-3 quarts boiling water

Method:

1. Add salt and boiling water in a large stockpot or brining container. Add the wines and broth. Juice the oranges and add the juice as well as the peels, garlic, onion, peppercorns, bay leaves and cloves. Stir until the salt is completely dissolved.
2. Place the turkey in it with the breast side down.
3. Place the turkey in brine in the refrigerator for at least 12 hours. There is nothing to worry if your turkey turns purple in color. In fact, it will taste even better.
4. Remove the turkey from the brine and pat it dry with paper towels. Rub oil over it. Brush soy sauce all over the turkey and rub it well into it.

5. Give a generous sprinkle of pepper. Lay the turkey on a rack in a big foil pan.
6. Stuff the inner hollow cavity (remove everything from the cavity) of turkey with onions, garlic and apple pieces.
7. Take 2 large sheets of foil. Fold one of its ends into a point. Place this point in between the legs of the turkey.
8. Brush oil on the foil that will touch the turkey while covering it. Fold the foil over the body of the turkey.
9. Operate the grill following the instructions of the manufacturer. Set the Kamado grill for smoking with the temperature at 500 ° F for about 30 minutes.
10. Place 3-6 mesquite or hickory wood chunks or wood chunks of your choice or 3-5 handfuls chips over the charcoal for smoking. Close the dome until you place the meat.
11. Place lava stone under the grill grates.
12. Place the turkey in the pan on the grill grate. Close the dome. Cook for 30 minutes.
13. Remove the turkey out from the grill and lower the temperature to 325 ° F.
14. Place a meat thermometer in the thickest part of the meat. Place the turkey back in the grill. Cover and cook until the temperature in the thermometer shows 165° F.
15. Remove the turkey from the grill and let it sit for 45 minutes. Unwrap the foil and serve.

Honey Pecan Chorizo Jalapeño Poppers

Ingredients:

- 32 medium jalapeños, halved, deseeded
- 1 package pork chorizo
- Deez nuts pecan rub, rub as required
- 2 packages standard cut bacon
- 2 blocks cream cheese (16 ounces each)

Method:

1. Place a skillet over medium heat. Add chorizo and sauté until cooked. Drain excess fat in the skillet. Add chorizo into a bowl. Add cream cheese and mix well.
2. Add nut pecan rub and mix well. Taste and add more of the rub if required.
3. Stuff this mixture into the halved jalapeños. Wrap each half with half a slice of bacon. Sprinkle some pecan rub on it.
4. Operate the grill following the instructions of the manufacturer. Set the Kamado grill for indirect cooking with the temperature at 275 ° F for about 15-20 minutes.
5. Place 3-6 mesquite or hickory wood chunks or wood chunks of your choice or 3-5 handfuls chips over the charcoal for smoking. Close the dome until you place the meat.
6. Place the poppers on the grill. Smoke for an hour or until the bacon is cooked.

Double Smoked Potatoes

Ingredients:

- 6 large baking potatoes, scrubbed, pat dried
- Coarse sea salt to taste
- Freshly ground black pepper to taste
- 3 tablespoons butter, melted
- 6 slices bacon, cut crosswise into ¼ inch slivers
- 2 scallions, chopped
- 3 cups cheese, shredded coarsely
- 10-12 tablespoons sour cream
- Smoked paprika to garnish
- Thin slices of butter to top (take cold butter and cut thin slices of it)

Method:

1. Operate the grill following the instructions of the manufacturer. Set the Kamado grill for smoking with the temperature at 400 ° F for about 15 minutes.
2. Place 3-6 wood chunks of your choice or 3-5 handfuls chips over the charcoal for smoking. Close the dome until you place the potatoes.
3. Prick all over the potatoes with a fork.
4. Brush the potatoes with some of the butter. Season with salt and pepper.
5. Place the potatoes on the grill. Cover with a dome. Smoke the potatoes until tender (it should be easily pierced with a bamboo skewer).
6. Meanwhile, place a skillet over medium heat. Add bacon. Cook until crisp. Drain excess fat. Set aside for a while.
7. When the potatoes are tender, remove and place on your cutting board. Halve the potatoes. Scoop out most of the cooked potato retaining the potato cases.
8. Place the scooped potatoes in a bowl. Mash until chunky in texture.
9. Add rest of the ingredients, some more salt, and pepper and mix well. Stuff this mixture into the cases of the potatoes.
10. Place a thin slice of butter over each of the stuffed potatoes. Sprinkle paprika over it.
11. Place it back on the grill. Cover the dome and cook until the top is brown or as per your liking.

Smoked Almonds

Ingredients:

- 2 cups whole almonds, unsalted
- Seasoned salt to taste
- 2 tablespoons hot sauce or to taste
- Pepper to taste

Method:

1. Operate the grill following the instructions of the manufacturer. Set the Kamado for smoking with the temperature at 200 ° F for about 15 minutes.
2. Place 3-6 wood chunks of your choice or 3-5 handfuls chips over the charcoal for smoking. Close the dome until you place the almonds.
3. Transfer the almonds on to a baking dish.
4. Place the dish on the grill. Close the dome. Smoke for about an hour or until dry. Stir every 15 minutes until dry.
5. Remove from the grill and cool completely. Store in an airtight container.

Smoked Mac and Cheese

Ingredients:

- 3 cups uncooked macaroni
- 1 ¾ cups milk
- ¾ teaspoon chipotle chili powder
- 1 cup parmesan cheese, shredded
- 4-5 cups cheddar cheese, shredded, divided
- ¾ stick butter
- 3 eggs, beaten
- Salt to taste
- Pepper to taste

Method:

1. Operate the grill following the instructions of the manufacturer. Set the Kamado for smoking with the temperature at 350 ° F for about 15 minutes.
2. Place 3-6 wood chunks of your choice or 3-5 handfuls chips over the charcoal for smoking. Close the dome until you place the baking dish.
3. Cook macaroni according to the instructions on the package until al dente. Drain.
4. Add butter to the macaroni and mix well. Add eggs, milk and chili powder and mix again. Add 2-3 cups cheddar cheese and stir. Transfer into a baking dish.
5. Sprinkle remaining cheddar cheese over it. Sprinkle Parmesan cheese rig on top of the cheddar cheese. Sprinkle salt and pepper over it.
6. Place the dish on the grill. Smoke for about 25 minutes.
7. Now raise the temperature to 350 ° F. Smoke for a few more minutes until brown on top.

Smoked Mango Macadamia Crisp

Ingredients:

- 10 cups fresh ripe mango, peeled, pitted, thinly sliced
- 4 tablespoons all-purpose flour
- 4 tablespoons candied ginger, minced
- ½ cup brown sugar or to taste
- Zest of 2 lemons, grated,
- Juice of 4 lemons

For the topping:

- ½ cup cold butter, chopped
- 1 cup macadamia nuts, coarsely chopped
- ½ cup all-purpose flour
- 1 cup shredded sweetened coconut
- 1 cup shortbread or butter cookies, crushed
- 1/8 teaspoon salt
- ½ cup firmly packed brown sugar
- 2 teaspoons ground cinnamon
- Whipped cream or vanilla ice cream to serve (optional)

Method:

1. Place mangoes in a glass bowl. Add ½ cup brown sugar, candied ginger, lemon juice and lemon zest and toss well. Add flour and mix well. Taste and adjust the brown sugar if required. Transfer into a cast iron skillet and set aside.
2. Add all the ingredients for the topping except cream into the food processor bowl and pulse until the mixture is coarse. Give short pulses only until the butter becomes smaller in size. Sprinkle this mixture over the mangoes in the skillet.
3. Operate the grill following the instructions of the manufacturer. Set the temperature between 245° F for about 25-30 minutes. Set for raised cooking.
4. Place 3-6 wood chunks of your choice or 3-5 handfuls chips over the charcoal for smoking. Close the dome until you place the skillet.

5. Place the skillet on the grill. Close the dome. Cook for about 45-60 minutes or until the top is golden brown in color.
6. Remove from the grill and cool for a while. Serve warm as it is or with ice cream or cream.

Chapter 7: Kamado Grill Roasting Recipes

Roasted Sweet Potatoes

Ingredients:

- 6 sweet potatoes

Method:

1. Operate the grill following the instructions of the manufacturer. Set the temperature for 300° F for about 25-30 minutes. Set for indirect cooking.
2. Place the sweet potatoes on the rack. Cook for 40-60 minutes. Rotate the sweet potatoes every 10-12 minutes until cooked.

Easy Roasted Whole Chicken

Ingredients:

- 1 whole chicken of about 3-4 pounds, clean the cavity, rinsed, pat dried
- 5 bay leaves
- 2 teaspoons whole peppercorns
- 2 lemons, halved
- 2 teaspoons whole cloves
- Kosher salt to taste

Method:

1. Stuff 2 halves of the lemon in the back of the cavity with the cut part of the lemon touching the chicken.
2. Also, stuff in the cavity, bay leaves, pepper, and cloves. Sprinkle salt. Stuff the remaining 2 halves of the lemon.
3. Close the chicken by trussing the chicken. Sprinkle some more salt and pepper on the outer surface of the chicken.
4. Operate the grill following the instructions of the manufacturer. Set the temperature for 360-380° F for about 25-30 minutes.
5. Place 3-6 mesquite or hickory wood chunks or wood chunks of your choice or 3-5 handfuls chips over the charcoal. Close the dome until you place the meat.
6. Roast for 1-1 ½ hours or until meat thermometer when inserted in the thickest portion of the meat shows 160-165 ° F. Rotate the chicken by 90 ° every 15 minutes.

Baby Dutch Yellow Potatoes with Roasted Hatch Chile Vinaigrette

Ingredients:

- 2 pounds Melissa's Baby Dutch yellow potatoes, halved
- 2 tablespoons extra virgin olive oil
- 2 onions, thinly sliced, caramelized
- Pepper to taste
- Salt to taste
- 2 cloves garlic, chopped
- ¾ pound Melissa's Hatch chiles, roasted

For vinaigrette:

- 1 cup salad oil
- 1/3 cup granulated sugar
- 1 clove garlic, chopped
- 1 1/3 cups seasoned rice vinegar
- 1/3-pound Melissa's Hatch chili, roasted
- Salt to taste
- Pepper to taste

Method:

1. Operate the grill following the instructions of the manufacturer. Set the Kamado grill for roasting with indirect cooking. Set the temperature at 350 ° F.
2. Add potatoes, oil, salt, garlic, and pepper into a bowl and toss well.
3. Transfer into a Paella pan. Place the pan on the grill. Roast for 25 minutes or until potatoes is tender.
4. Remove the potatoes from the grill and set aside to cool.
5. To make the vinaigrette: Add all the ingredients except oil into a blender. With the motor of the blender running, slowly add oil in a thin stream until the mixture emulsifies. Add more oil if required. Taste and adjust the seasonings if necessary.
6. To make salad: Add potatoes, caramelized, onions, and roasted chilies into a serving bowl. Pour as much dressing as required. Toss well and serve.

Lager Roasted Vegetables

Ingredients:

- 2 heads broccoli, chopped into florets
- 2 green bell peppers, deseeded, cut into ½ inch wide strips
- 1 red bell pepper, deseeded, cut into ½ inch wide strips
- 1 yellow bell pepper, deseeded, cut into ½ inch wide strips
- 25 cloves garlic
- 2 heads cauliflower, chopped into florets
- 2 sprigs rosemary, chopped
- 2 sprigs oregano, chopped
- 2 sprigs thyme, chopped
- 2 sprigs parsley, chopped
- 12 ounces lager beer
- Freshly cracked pepper to taste
- Kosher salt to taste
- 2 cups parmesan cheese, grated
- 4 tablespoons butter, unsalted

Method:

1. Add all the ingredients except cheese and butter into a zip lock bag. Shake the bag until the vegetables are well coated with the remaining ingredients. Refrigerate overnight.
2. Operate the grill following the instructions of the manufacturer. Set the Kamado grill for roasting with indirect cooking. Set the temperature at 425 ° F.
3. Empty the contents of the zip lock bag on to the roasting accessory or paella pan.
4. Place the pan on the grill and roast for 30-40 minutes. Stir a couple of times while it is roasting.
5. Add butter and mix well. Roast for 10 minutes.
6. Remove from the grill and mix well. Sprinkle cheese over it and serve immediately.

Roasted Beet Soup

Ingredients:

- ½ small celeriac along with a few of its greens, cubed
- 1 red onion, quartered
- 12 large beetroots
- 1 carrot, peeled, cubed
- 6 tablespoons butter, melted
- 6 cups vegetable stock
- 6 tablespoons balsamic vinegar
- 1 cup crème Fraiche
- 4 bay leaves
- 4 tablespoons horseradish puree
- Fresh horseradish, as required, grated
- 2 small containers watercress

Method:

1. Operate the grill following the instructions of the manufacturer. Set the Kamado grill for roasting.
2. Place onions, bay leaves, celery leaves, celeriac, carrot, and celery leaves on an aluminum foil. Pour melted butter over it. Wrap the foil.
3. Place the beets directly on the charcoal. Roast for 35-45 minutes depending on the size of the beets. Turn the beets around every 10 minutes. Place the wrapped vegetables on the beets during the last 20-25 minutes of cooking. Do not place it directly on charcoal.
4. When done, remove the vegetables from the grill. Cool for a while. Unwrap the foil and discard the bay leaves.
5. When cool enough to handle, peel the beets and chop into smaller pieces.
6. Add beets, broth, horseradish puree, vegetables, vinegar, salt, and pepper into a blender and blend until smooth.
7. Pour into a saucepan. Place the saucepan over medium heat and bring to the boil.
8. Ladle into soup bowls. Drizzle some crème Fraiche. Garnish with horseradish and watercress and serve.

Easy Roasted Potatoes

Ingredients:

- 6 whole potatoes
- 2 tablespoons olive oil
- Salt to taste
- Pepper to taste
- 2 teaspoons granulated garlic

Method:

1. Rub potatoes with oil. Operate the grill following the instructions of the manufacturer. Set the Kamado grill for indirect cooking. Place the plate setter below the grill grate. Set the temperature at 350-450 ° F.
2. Place the potatoes on the grill grate.
3. Season with granulated garlic, salt, and pepper.
4. Close the dome. Roast for about 25-30 minutes or until the potatoes are tender.
5. Serve hot.

Garlic, Herb and Lemon Roasted Leg of Lamb

Ingredients:

- 4 pounds leg of lamb, trimmed
- ¼ cup fresh thyme, finely chopped
- ½ cup fresh oregano, finely chopped
- ½ cup fresh rosemary, finely chopped
- 2 tablespoons garlic, chopped
- 2 teaspoons lemon zest
- Pepper to taste
- 2 teaspoons kosher salt or to taste
- ¼ cup lemon juice
- 2 bulbs garlic (halve the whole garlic along with its skin)
- 2 sticks butter, unsalted, at room temperature
- ½ cup olive oil
- 2 lemons, halved

Method:

1. Operate the grill following the instructions of the manufacturer. Set the Kamado grill for roasting with indirect cooking. Set the temperature at 375 ° F.
2. Close the lamb by trussing the lamb and placing it in a plastic container.
3. Add butter, fresh herbs, oil, lemon zest, spices and lemon juice into a bowl. Mix well. Remove about ½ cup of the mixture into a bowl and set it aside.
4. Sprinkle salt all over the lamb. Spread the remaining herb mixture all over the lamb and rub it well into the lamb. Place lamb in the roasting accessory.
5. Place the lemon halves in the roasting accessory with the cut side facing the bottom of the pan. Also, place the garlic bulb halves with the cut side facing up.
6. Place the roasting accessory on the grill and roast for about an hour or until a meat thermometer shows 130 ° F.
7. Baste the lamb with its drippings that are collected in the roasting accessory. Do this every 20-30 minutes.
8. Pour rest of the herb mixture on the lamb during the last 10 minutes of roasting. Spread it all over the lamb.
9. Remove the lamb from the grill and place on a serving platter. Also, remove the garlic and lemon halves and squeeze its juices all over the lamb.

Salt Seared Lamb Chop with Fresh Mint Sauce

Ingredients:

- 2 racks lamb chops
- 2-3 cloves garlic, peeled, smashed
- 2 tablespoons grape seed oil

For mint sauce:

- 2 cups fresh mint leaves
- 3 tablespoons confectioner's sugar
- 2 cups apple cider vinegar
- 2 teaspoons fresh lemon juice

Method:

1. To make the mint sauce: Add all the ingredients of mint sauce into a blender and pulse for a few seconds until mint leaves are chopped. Transfer into a bowl and refrigerate until use. While serving, serve it either room temperature or slightly warm.
2. Operate the grill following the instructions of the manufacturer. Set the Kamado grill for roasting with indirect cooking. Set the temperature to 350 ° F and preheat for 20 minutes. Now raise the temperature to 450 ° F for 20 minutes.
3. Place a salt block on top of the plate setter.
4. Pat dry the lamb chops. Chop into individual chops if you are using a rack of lamb chops.
5. Rub garlic all over the lamb chops. Brush grape seed oil all over the lamb chops.
6. Place the lamb chops on the salt block and roast until meat thermometer when inserted in the thickest portion of the meat shows 140 ° F.
7. Remove from the grill and cover with foil. Let it sit for 10 minutes.
8. Serve with mint sauce.

Prime Rib Roast

Ingredients:

- 1 rib roast of beef or bison
- 2 tablespoons olive oil
- 2 tablespoons garlic, minced
- 5-6 tablespoons rub of your choice

Method:

1. Remove the roast from the refrigerator and bring to room temperature.
2. Place roast on a large foil sheet. Sprinkle garlic and seasoning over it. Wrap with foil and refrigerate for 12-24 hours. Remove from the refrigerator an hour before cooking.
3. Operate the grill following the instructions of the manufacturer. Set the Kamado grill for roasting with indirect cooking. Set the temperature to 500 ° F and preheat for 20 minutes.
4. Place a cast iron griddle on the grill. Unwrap and place meat on the griddle.
5. Braise with the juices remaining in the foil. Roast for 10 minutes on each side.
6. Now lower the temperature to 200 ° F and cook for 30-40 minutes or until meat thermometer when inserted in the thickest portion of the meat shows 140 ° F.
7. Remove from the grill and let it rest for 15 minutes before serving.

The Perfect Roasted Turkey

Ingredients:

- 1 whole turkey of 10-12 pounds
- 2 stalks celery, chopped
- Turkey rub of your choice, as required
- 2 whole onions, halved
- Chicken broth or wine or water, as required

Method:

1. Operate the grill following the instructions of the manufacturer. Set the Kamado grill for roasting with indirect cooking. Set the temperature at 375 ° F.
2. Place a drip pan on the bottom shelf.
3. Place turkey on a vertical poultry roaster or V-rack. Place it in the drip pan. Also, place onion and celery in the drip pan. Pour water or broth or wine to fill the drip pan.
4. Roast for 2 ½ - 3 hours or until meat thermometer when inserted in the breast portion of the meat shows 160 ° F.
5. Remove from the grill and let it rest for 15 minutes before serving.
6. Pour the drippings remaining in the drip pan over the turkey and serve.

Roasted Pears

Ingredients:

- 8 large pears, preferably with stems, halved lengthwise
- 10 tablespoons butter, at room temperature
- 10 tablespoons graham cracker crumbs or ground hazelnuts
- 1 teaspoon ground cinnamon
- 1 teaspoon ground cloves
- 2 teaspoons vanilla extract
- Juice of a lemon
- 10 tablespoons brown sugar
- 1 teaspoon lemon zest, grated
- ½ teaspoon nutmeg, grated
- 2 tablespoons rum
- 2 cups Poire Williams (Pear Brandy)

Method:

1. Take a melon scooper and scoop the core of the pears. You should be left with pear cases with a cavity in the center that can be stuffed with filling.
2. Brush scored part of the pear with lemon juice.
3. Add butter and brown sugar into a bowl and beat until fluffy. Add graham cracker crumbs, nutmeg, cinnamon, cloves, lemon zest and vanilla and beat until well combined.
4. Fill this mixture in the pears in the cavity of the core.
5. Place the stuffed pears in a greased disposable aluminum foil pan.
6. Operate the grill following the instructions of the manufacturer. Set the Kamado grill for roasting with indirect cooking. Set the temperature at 275 ° F.
7. Add 4-6 apple or peach wood chunks in it.
8. Place the disposable pan on the grill. Close the dome of the grill.
9. Roast until the pears are soft and brown. It should take 45-60 minutes. But keep a check.
10. Remove the pears from the disposable pan and place on a fireproof platter.

11. Meanwhile, place a saucepan over medium heat. Add Poire Williams and let it warm up. Remove from heat.
12. Light a matchstick and touch the flame to the brandy. It will catch fire. Pour the brandy along with the flame over the pears.
13. Serve immediately.

Chapter 8: Kamado Grill Steaming Recipes

Seafood Paella

Ingredients:

For fish stock:

- 1-pound small rock fish or fish bones
- 2 ripe tomatoes, quartered
- 6-7 cups water
- 6 mussels
- 1 medium red onion, chopped
- A pinch saffron strands (optional)
- 2 teaspoons olive oil

For the tomato sauce:

- 1 medium red onion, chopped
- 2 cloves garlic, minced
- 2 tablespoons olive oil
- 26-28 ounces canned, crushed tomatoes
- A little sugar (optional)

For paella:

- 2 cups paella rice
- ¼ pound squid rings
- 18-20 green prawns
- 18-20 mussels
- Crab (optional)

Method:

1. To make fish stock: Place a stockpot over medium heat. Add oil. When the oil is heated, add onion and sauté until golden brown.
2. Add rest of the ingredients of stock and bring to the boil.
3. Lower heat to medium low and simmer for 1-½ hours.
4. Strain and use as much as required for paella.
5. To make tomato sauce: Meanwhile, place a skillet over medium heat. Add oil. When the oil is heated, add onions and sauté until golden brown. Set aside half the onions in a bowl.
6. Add garlic to the skillet and sauté for 2-3 minutes. Add tomatoes and mix well.
7. Lower heat and simmer for 20-30 minutes. Add sugar to taste only if the sauce is sour. Remove from heat.
8. Operate the grill following the instructions of the manufacturer. Set the Kamado grill for indirect cooking. Set the temperature at 375 ° F.
9. Place a diffuser plate. Add the onion that was set-aside into the paella pan. Add tomato sauce and place the paella pan on the diffuser plate. Let it cook for 5 minutes.
10. Add all the seafood and rice and mix well. Add half-cup stock. Cook until the stock is absorbed. Add more stock, a little at a time, cook until it is absorbed.
11. Now close the dome and cook for 5 minutes.
12. Serve.

Chicken and Sausage Paella

Ingredients:

- 3 Italian sausages, cut into 1-inch pieces
- 3-5 chicken thighs or breast pieces
- 1 ½ pounds shrimp, peeled, deveined
- 3 onions, chopped
- 1 ½ cans (28 ounces each) diced tomatoes
- 1 ½ cups white wine
- 4 ½ cups chicken broth
- 2 medium red bell peppers, deseeded, chopped
- 3-4 bay leaves
- 1 ½ cups frozen peas, thawed
- 3 cups Arborio rice
- 3 tablespoons garlic, minced
- 1 tablespoon olive oil

Method:

1. Operate the grill following the instructions of the manufacturer. Set the Kamado grill for indirect cooking. Set the temperature at 325-350 ° F.
2. Place a diffuser plate. Place the paella pan on the diffuser plate. Add oil. When the oil is heated, add chicken and sausages and sauté until brown. Remove on to a plate and set aside to add along with rice.
3. Add onions and garlic to the paella pan and sauté until golden brown. Add tomatoes and stir.
4. Now lower the temperature to 225-250 ° F.
5. Add rest of the ingredients except peas and shrimp and stir.
6. Cover the dome. Cook for about 20 minutes. Add shrimp and peas.
7. Cover and cook until all the broth is absorbed and rice is tender. In case the rice is not cooked, and broth is absorbed, add a little more broth.

Steamed Broccoli

Ingredients:

- 1 large broccoli, chop into florets of about 1-1 ½ inches each
- 1 cup water or broth or wine
- 4 tablespoons olive oil
- Salt to taste
- Pepper to taste
- 2 teaspoons butter (optional)

Method:

1. Add all the ingredients into a zip lock bag. Seal the bag and shake until the broccoli is well coated with the remaining mixture. Refrigerate until use.
2. Take a heavy-duty foil sheet or take 2 foil sheets. Lift the edges to shape like a bowl. Transfer the contents of the zip lock bag and seal the foil completely.
3. Operate the grill following the instructions of the manufacturer. Set the Kamado grill for direct cooking.
4. Place the foil packet directly on the charcoal. Steam for 10 minutes.
5. Remove from the grill, unwrap and serve immediately.

Warm Cauliflower Salad

Ingredients:

- 2 ½ tablespoons olive oil
- 2 tablespoons water
- 1 teaspoon onion powder or granulated onion
- ½ teaspoon salt
- 1 tablespoon lemon juice
- 1 small red onion, thinly sliced
- ¼ cup black olives pitted, halved
- 3 -4 cup cauliflower florets of about 1- 1 ½ inches each
- 1 teaspoon dried basil
- ½ teaspoon dried oregano
- 1 clove garlic, peeled, crushed
- 1 tablespoon mayonnaise or more if required
- 2 tablespoons fresh parsley, chopped

Method:

1. Take a heavy-duty foil sheet or take 2 foil sheets. Lift the edges to shape like a bowl. Place cauliflower in it and pour water and seal the foil completely.
2. Operate the grill following the instructions of the manufacturer. Set the Kamado for direct cooking.
3. Place the foil packet directly on the charcoal. Steam for 10 minutes.
4. Remove from the grill, unwrap and transfer to a serving bowl.
5. Add rest of the ingredients and toss well. Taste and adjust the seasoning and mayonnaise if desired.
6. Serve immediately.

Steamed Potatoes with Shallots, Lemon and Thyme

Ingredients:

- ¾ pound small red potatoes (1 ½ -2 inches diameter), halved
- ¾ pound small Yukon gold potatoes (1 ½ -2 inches diameter), halved
- 2 tablespoons extra virgin olive oil
- 1 medium shallot, chopped
- Freshly ground pepper to taste
- Kosher salt to taste
- 2 tablespoons fresh lemon juice or to taste
- 1 tablespoon fresh thyme leaves, finely minced

Method:

1. Add potatoes, shallots, lemon juice, oil, thyme, salt, and pepper into a bowl and toss well.
2. Take 2-3 large heavy-duty foil sheets or take 2-3 sets of 2 foil sheets. Lift the edges to shape like a bowl. Divide the contents of the bowl into the foil and seal the foil completely.
3. Operate the grill following the instructions of the manufacturer. Set the Kamado grill for direct cooking.
4. Place the foil packets on the grill grate. Steam for 20 minutes. Turn the packets by about 90 degrees every 10 minutes.
5. Remove from the grill and cool for a few minutes. Unwrap and transfer into a serving bowl.
6. Taste and adjust the seasoning if desired.
7. Garnish with some more thyme if desired and serve immediately.

Steamed Clams

Ingredients:

- 2 pounds fresh clams
- 1 large onion, sliced
- 2 tablespoons butter

Method:

1. Operate the grill following the instructions of the manufacturer. Set the Kamado grill for direct cooking.
2. Place the clams on the grill grate. Steam for 15-20 minutes. The clams get steamed in their shells. Slowly the clams will begin to open up. The clams are ready when they have opened. Discard the unopened ones.
3. Meanwhile, place a skillet over medium heat. Add butter. When the butter melts, add onion and sauté until light brown. Remove from heat.
4. Dip the clams in the onion-butter dip and serve.

Thyme Smoked Mussels

Ingredients:

- 2 pounds rope grown mussels, washed, debearded
- 2 banana shallots, finely chopped
- Juice of a lemon
- 1 teaspoon lemon zest, grated
- ½ small bunch flat leaf parsley, chopped
- 1 clove garlic, peeled, finely chopped
- Olive oil, as required
- 4-8 sprigs dried thyme

Method:

1. Operate the grill following the instructions of the manufacturer. Set the Kamado grill for direct cooking.
2. Add mussels into a bowl. Drizzle oil over it. Toss well.
3. Place thyme sprigs directly on the charcoal. Place the mussels on the grill.
4. Place the mussels on the grill grate. Steam for 15-20 minutes. The mussels get steamed in their shells. Slowly the mussels will begin to open up. The mussels are ready when they have opened. Discard the unopened ones.
5. Meanwhile, add rest of the ingredients into a bowl and toss well.
6. Add steamed mussels into the bowl and toss well.
7. Serve.

Lemon Dill Salmon Packets

Ingredients:

- 6 salmon fillets (6 ounces each)
- 1 ½ tablespoons butter, softened
- Salt to taste
- Pepper to taste
- 6 cloves garlic, sliced
- 1 medium onion, sliced
- 6 fresh dill sprigs
- 1 large lemon, sliced
- 2 tablespoons fresh basil, minced

Method:

1. Take 6 large heavy-duty foil sheets or take 6 sets of 2 foil sheets. Divide the butter among the 6 foils and place in the center. Season with salt and pepper. Divide and place rest of the ingredients over it and seal the foil completely.
2. Operate the grill following the instructions of the manufacturer. Set the Kamado grill for direct cooking.
3. Place the foil packets on the grill. Steam for 8-10 minutes or until it flakes easily when pierced with a fork.
4. Remove from the grill. Cool for a couple of minutes and serve.

BBQ Hot Dog and Potatoes

Ingredients:

- 1 ½ packages (20 ounces each) refrigerated red potato wedges
- 2 small onions, cut into wedges
- ¾ cup BBQ sauce
- 6 hot dogs
- 1/3 cup cheddar cheese, shredded

Method:

1. Take 6 large heavy-duty foil sheets or take 6 sets of 2 large foil sheets. Divide the potato wedges among the 6 foils and place in the center. Place a hot dog over the potatoes on each of the foils. Divide the onion and place on the potatoes. Sprinkle cheese over it. Spoon some BBQ sauce over it. Seal the foil completely.
2. Operate the grill following the instructions of the manufacturer. Set the Kamado grill for direct cooking.
3. Place the foil packets on the grill. Cover the grill. Steam for 10-15 minutes.
4. When done, remove the packets and cool for 3-4 minutes

Cheese Hash Browns

Ingredients:

- 1 ½ packages (28 ounces each) frozen hash browns, thawed
- 12 ounces bacon strips, cooked, chopped
- Pepper to taste
- Salt to taste
- 2 cups cheddar cheese, divided
- Hard boiled eggs to serve, as required (optional)
- Pico de gallo

Method:

1. Add potatoes into a bowl. Add half the cheese, salt, pepper and bacon.
5. Take 6 large heavy-duty foil sheets or take 6 sets of 2 foil sheets. Divide the potato mixture among the 6 foils and place in the center. Seal the foil completely.
6. Operate the grill following the instructions of the manufacturer. Set the Kamado grill for direct cooking.
2. Place the foil packets on the grill. Steam for 8-10 minutes.
3. When done, remove the packets and cool for 3-4 minutes. Garnish with remaining cheese.
4. Serve with eggs and pico de gallo.

Scallops, Asparagus, and Artichoke Gratin

Ingredients:

- ¾ pound sea scallops
- ¼ cup shallots, finely chopped
- 1 cup cream
- ¾ cup parmesan cheese, shaved, divided
- Pepper to taste
- Salt to taste
- ¼ teaspoon crushed red pepper
- 1 can (15 ounces) artichoke hearts, drained
- 4 tablespoons butter, unsalted, butter
- 3 tablespoons all-purpose flour
- ½ cup milk
- ¼ teaspoon lemon zest, grated
- 1-pound asparagus, trimmed, blanched
- ¼ cup bacon, cooked, crumbled
- 2 tablespoons panko bread crumbs

Method:

1. Operate the grill following the instructions of the manufacturer. Set the Kamado grill for baking with the temperature at 350 ° F for about 25-30 minutes. Set for direct cooking.
2. Add 4-6 wood chunks in it.
3. Place a cast iron skillet over the grill. Add half the butter. When it melts, add scallops and cook until light brown and nearly opaque. Turn it once after a few minutes of cooking. Transfer scallops on to a plate. Set aside.
4. Add remaining butter to the skillet. When butter melts, add shallots and sauté until tender. Add flour and sauté until fragrant.
5. Slowly pour the milk and cream into the skillet, stirring constantly. Keep stirring until the mixture is thick.
6. Add cheese, salt, pepper, red pepper and lemon zest and mix well. Add artichoke hearts and asparagus and mix well. Sprinkle breadcrumbs and bacon.
7. Cover the dome. Steam for 8-10 minutes and serve.

Corn on the Cob

Ingredients:

- 6 ears shucked corn
- ½ cup parmesan cheese, shredded
- Salt to taste
- Pepper to taste
- 1/3 cup butter or olive oil
- 1 teaspoon dried rosemary leaves
- 6 ice cubes

Method:

1. Operate the grill following the instructions of the manufacturer. Set the Kamado grill for direct cooking with the temperature at 350 ° F for about 25-30 minutes.
2. Add 4-6 wood chunks in it.
3. Take 6 large heavy-duty foil sheets or take 6 sets of 2 foil sheets. Place corn in the center of each foil. Brush butter over it. Sprinkle rosemary, salt, and pepper over the corn. Sprinkle cheese. Place a cube of ice on each. Seal the foil completely like a tent.
4. Place the foil packets on the charcoal. Steam for 20 minutes.
5. When done, remove the packets and cool for 3-4 minutes.

Breakfast Burritos

Ingredients:

- ½ pound bacon, cubed
- ½ pound cheese, shredded
- 1-pound frozen hash browns
- ½ pound sausage, crumbled
- 6 eggs
- 6 large flour tortillas
- Toppings and salsa of your choice

Method:

1. Operate the grill following the instructions of the manufacturer. Set the Kamado grill for direct cooking with the temperature at 250 ° F for about 10 minutes.
2. Add 4-6 wood chunks in it.
3. Place the Dutch oven on the grill. Add bacon and sausage and cook until brown.
4. Add hash browns and stir. Cover the Dutch oven. Close the dome. Cook for 10 minutes.
5. Pour eggs into the Dutch oven and stir. Cover the Dutch oven and close the dome. Cook for 5 minutes or until the eggs are set.
6. Remove from the grill. Add cheese and stir.
7. Warm the tortillas according to the instructions on the package. Place tortillas on your work area. Spoon some of the sausage fillings. Top with toppings. Wrap and serve.

Steamed Apples

Ingredients:

- 4 apples, cored but leave the bottom intact
- ½ cup nuts of your choice, chopped
- 2 teaspoons butter
- ½ cup dried fruit
- 2 teaspoons sugar
- 4 teaspoons ground cinnamon

Method:

1. Stuff the cored cavity of the apples with a mixture of dried fruits and nuts. Press well.
2. Sprinkle a mixture of cinnamon and sugar. Place a little butter on top.
3. Wrap each of the apples in heavy-duty sheets of foil or double-layered foil.
4. Operate the grill following the instructions of the manufacturer. Set the Kamado grill for direct cooking.
5. Place the foil packet directly on the charcoal. The filled portion should be upright. Steam for 12-18 minutes, according to the way you like the apples steamed.
6. Remove from the grill, unwrap and transfer to a serving bowl.

Applesauce Gingerbread Cake

Ingredients:

- 1 ½ packages gingerbread cake mix
- 1 ½ cans (14 ounces each) applesauce

Method:

1. Operate the grill following the instructions of the manufacturer. Set the Kamado grill for indirect cooking.
2. Take a cast iron Dutch oven or skillet and add applesauce into it.
3. Sprinkle cake mix over it. Do not mix.
4. Cover the skillet and cover the dome of the grill. Steam for about 20-30 minutes.
5. Remove from the grill and cool for a few minutes.
6. Serve warm.

Glazed Peaches

Ingredients:

- 6 peaches, pitted, quartered
- 3 tablespoons butter
- 5 tablespoons brown sugar
- 2 teaspoons ground cinnamon

Method:

1. Operate the grill following the instructions of the manufacturer. Set the Kamado grill with the temperature at 350 ° F for about 25-30 minutes. Set for direct cooking.
2. Add 4-6 wood chunks into the grill.
3. Add all the ingredients into a bowl and mix well.
4. Take a heavy-duty foil sheet or take 2 foil sheets. Lift the edges to shape like a bowl. Transfer the peach mixture into it. Seal it completely.
5. Place the foil packet directly on the charcoal. Steam for 10-12 minutes.
6. Remove from the grill, unwrap and serve.

Chapter 9: Kamado Grill Braising Recipes

Pot Roast

Ingredients:

- 1 pot roast
- Freshly ground pepper to taste
- Salt to taste
- 4 potatoes, cubed
- 2 carrots, peeled, cubed
- 2 stalks celery, chopped
- Beef broth, as required
- 2 medium onions, quartered
- 5-6 tablespoons brown gravy mix

Method:

1. Operate the grill following the instructions of the manufacturer. Set the Kamado grill for direct cooking. Set the temperature at 350 ° F.
2. Sprinkle roast pot salt and pepper. Place on the grill and sear for a few minutes on all the sides.
3. Now remove the roast and place in a cast iron Dutch oven. Add the vegetables. Pour enough broth to nearly cover the roast. Pour brown gravy mix. Cover the Dutch oven.
4. Place the Dutch oven on the top rack. Cover the dome of the grill. Cook for 4-6 hours depending on how big the roast is.
5. Check the broth after 3-4 hours of cooking. Add more if needed.
6. Serve in soup bowls.

Authentic Irish Stew

Ingredients:

- 3 cups water
- 5 bay leaves
- 2 medium onions, chopped
- 10 carrots, cut into rounds
- 6 stalks celery, sliced
- 10 cloves garlic, chopped
- 2 teaspoons fresh rosemary, minced
- 21 ounces beef stock
- Salt to taste
- Pepper to taste
- 3 tablespoons olive oil
- 3 pounds lamb cut into 2-inch chunks
- 6 stalks chives, chopped
- 5 large Idaho potatoes, cubed
- 2 ½ cups mushrooms, sliced
- 2 teaspoons fresh thyme
- 1 ½ cups flour
- 1 ½ bottles (14.9 ounces each) Guinness Stout

Method:

1. Operate the grill following the instructions of the manufacturer. Set the Kamado grill for indirect cooking. Set the temperature at 225 ° F.
2. Place the heat deflector with the ceramic plate in bottom position in the grill. Place the grill grate on top.
3. Add 4-6 apple or peach wood chunks in it.
4. Add all the ingredient of the stew into a cast iron Dutch oven. Do not cover the lid of the Dutch oven.
5. Place the Dutch oven on the grill. Cover the dome of the grill. Cook for 1 ½ - 2 ½ hours or until meat is tender.
6. Check the broth after an hour of cooking. Add more if needed.
7. If the stew is watery, then uncover during the last 15-20 minutes of cooking.
8. Serve in bowls.

Smokey Mountain Brunswick Stew

Ingredients:

- 1 whole chicken of about 2 ½ -3 ½ pounds
- 3 medium onions, chopped
- 6 cups chicken broth
- 3 tablespoons Worcestershire sauce
- 24 ounces corn kernels
- 6 cloves, minced
- 2 Andouille sausages
- 1 large bell pepper, chopped
- 1 ½ cans (14.5 ounces each) diced tomatoes
- 24 ounces BBQ sauce
- 24 ounces butter beans
- 3 bottles beer

Method:

1. Operate the grill following the instructions of the manufacturer. Set the Kamado grill for indirect cooking. Set the temperature at 275 ° F.
2. Place the heat deflector with the ceramic plate in bottom position in the grill. Place the grill grate on top.
3. Add 4-6 apple or peach wood chunks in it.
4. Place the chicken stand in the grill and pour one bottle of beer in it. Place the chicken on the stand. Roast for 2 ½ - 3 hours. Add more beer after about 2 hours of cooking.
5. Add rest of the ingredients except Andouille sausage of the stew into a cast iron Dutch oven. Place the Dutch oven on your stovetop and simmer for a while.
6. Place the sausages on the grill during the last 30 minutes of roasting the chicken.
7. When the chicken and sausage is done, remove from the grill and place on your cutting board. When cool enough to handle, shred the chicken with a pair of forks. Chop the sausages into bite size pieces.

8. Add chicken and sausages into the Dutch oven. Transfer the Dutch oven from the stovetop to the grill.
9. Add remaining beer and stir.
10. Do not cover the lid of the Dutch oven.
11. Place the Dutch oven on the grill. Cover the dome of the grill.
12. Lower the temperature of the grill to 250 ° F. Cook for 1 ½ - 2 ½ hours or until the stew is thickened.
13. Serve in bowls with cornbread.

Hobo Stew

Ingredients:

- 2 pounds ground beef
- 2 cans (15 ounces each) whole peeled tomatoes
- 2 cups water
- 30 ounces mixed vegetables
- 4 ½ cups uncooked elbow macaroni
- Salt to taste
- Pepper to taste

Method:

1. Operate the grill following the instructions of the manufacturer. Set the Kamado grill for indirect cooking. Set the temperature at 225 ° F.
2. Place the heat deflector with the ceramic plate in bottom position in the grill.
3. Add wood chunks in it. Place the grill grate on top.
4. Place a cast iron Dutch oven on the grate. Add beef and cook until brown. Drain off excess fat. Add rest of the ingredient of the stew into the Dutch oven. Cover the Dutch oven.
5. Place the Dutch oven on the grill. Cover the dome of the grill. Cook for 1 ½ - 2 ½ hours or until macaroni is al dente.

Braised Chicken

Ingredients:

- 8 chicken thighs
- A handful rosemary, chopped
- A handful thyme, chopped
- 1 tablespoon garlic, minced
- 7-8 tablespoons mustard
- 2 ½ cups sherry
- 2-2 ½ cups chicken broth

Method:

1. Operate the grill following the instructions of the manufacturer. Set the Kamado grill for direct cooking. Set the temperature at 300 ° F.
2. Place chicken on the grill and sear for a few minutes on all the sides.
3. Transfer the chicken from the grill into a cast iron Dutch oven or pan. Sear for a few more minutes. Remove the chicken and set aside.
4. Add garlic to the pan. Sauté until fragrant. Add fresh herbs and sauté until fragrant. Add the seared chicken, mustard, and sherry. When the liquid in the pan is reduced to 1/3 the original quantity, add chicken broth and stir.
5. Simmer until the sauce is thickened.
6. Serve hot.

Beer Chicken

Ingredients:

- 1 whole chicken of 3-5 pounds
- Few slices lemon
- 12-15 ounces beer
- 12 cloves garlic, peeled
- 2 sprigs fresh oregano
- 2 sprigs fresh rosemary
- Salt to taste
- 7-8 tablespoons poultry rub of your choice

Method:

1. Operate the grill following the instructions of the manufacturer. Set the Kamado grill for indirect cooking. Set the temperature at 350 - 400 ° F.
2. Place the heat deflector with the ceramic plate in bottom position in the grill. Place the grill grate on top.
3. Season the chicken with a generous amount of salt. Then rub the chicken with poultry rub. Stuff cavity of the chicken with garlic and herbs.
4. Add 4-6 apple or peach wood chunks in it.
5. Place the chicken stand in the grill and pour beer into it. Place the chicken on the stand. Roast for 1 to 2 hours or until a meat thermometer shows 150 ° F.
6. When done, remove from the grill and let it sit for 10-15 minutes before serving.

Apple and Root Beer Baked Beans

Ingredients:

- 3 bacon strips, chopped
- 2 cans (16 ounces each) baked beans
- 10.5 ounces canned apple pie filling
- ½ teaspoon ancho chili pepper (optional)
- 6 ounces root beer
- ½ cup smoked cheddar cheese, shredded

Method:

1. Operate the grill following the instructions of the manufacturer. Set the Kamado grill for indirect cooking. Set the temperature at 275 ° F.
2. Place the heat deflector with the ceramic plate in bottom position in the grill. Place the grill grate on top.
3. Add 4-6 apple or peach wood chunks in it.
4. Place Dutch oven on the grill. Add bacon and cook until crisp. Remove bacon with a slotted spoon and discard the fat that is remaining in the pan. Add bacon back into the Dutch oven.
5. Add rest of the ingredients except cheese into the Dutch oven. Stir well. Cover the Dutch oven. Cover the dome of the grill. Cook for about 25-30 minutes.
6. Add cheese and stir. Serve right away.

Dutch Oven-Braised Beef and Summer Vegetables

Ingredients:

For beef:

- 12 garlic cloves, minced
- 4 tablespoons olive oil
- 1 teaspoon pepper powder
- ¼ cup fresh rosemary, chopped
- 2 teaspoons kosher salt
- 4 pounds beef chuck roast

For the vegetables:

- 2 pints cherry tomatoes, discard stems
- 2 onions, cut into 6 wedges each
- 1-pound baby zucchinis, trimmed,
- 4 tablespoons butter
- 4 ears corn, cleaned, cut into thirds
- 1-pound green beans, trimmed, cut in half
- 1 ½ pounds thin skinned potatoes (of about 1-inch diameter)
- 6 cups chicken broth, divided

Method:

1. For beef: Add garlic, oil, rosemary, pepper, and salt into a bowl and mix well. Rub this mixture all over the beef. Transfer into a zip lock bag. Seal and refrigerate until use. It can be refrigerated up to 2 days. You can also freeze if desired.
2. For vegetables: Add corn, tomatoes, and onions in another zip lock bag. Add zucchini and beans into a third zip lock bag. Refrigerate until use. It can be refrigerated up to 2 days.
3. Operate the grill following the instructions of the manufacturer. Set the Kamado grill for indirect cooking. Set the temperature at 300-350° F.
4. Place the heat deflector with the ceramic plate in bottom position in the grill. Place the grill grate on top.

5. Add 4-6 apple or peach wood chunks in it.
6. Place a cast iron Dutch oven on the grill. Add butter. When butter melts, add beef and cook until brown. Flip the side and add 4 cups broth. Cover the Dutch oven with its lid. Cover the dome of the grill. Cook for 1-2 hours.
7. Flip the beef again. Add remaining broth, the bag of tomato mixture and potatoes.
8. Cover the Dutch oven with its lid. Cover the dome of the grill. Cook for 1 hour.
9. Flip the beef again. Add more broth if required and the bag of beans mixture.
10. Cover the Dutch oven with its lid. Cover the dome of the grill. Cook for about 20 minutes or until the meat is tender.
11. Add salt and pepper to taste. Stir and serve.

Root Beer Braised Ribs

Ingredients:

- 3 pounds pork spare ribs

For the rub:

- 1 ½ teaspoons Hungarian paprika
- 1 ½ teaspoons pepper powder
- 1 ½ teaspoons salt

For braising:

- 2 medium red onions, minced
- 1 ½ teaspoons whole cumin seeds, crushed
- 5 bay leaves
- 18 ounces root beer
- 3 sprigs fresh rosemary
- 1 ½ inches ginger, peeled, minced
- ½ teaspoon hot Hungarian paprika
- ½ teaspoon ground cinnamon
- 1 ½ cups chicken or beef broth
- 5 sprigs fresh thyme

Method:

1. Mix together the ingredients of rub into a bowl. Mix well. Rub this mixture over the pork spare ribs.
2. Operate the grill following the instructions of the manufacturer. Set the Kamado grill for direct cooking. Set the temperature at 275 ° F.
3. Place a Dutch oven on the grill. Place spareribs in the Dutch oven and sear for a few minutes on all the sides.
4. Transfer the spareribs on to a plate and set aside.
5. Discard most of the fat that is remaining in the oven.

6. Add onions and sauté until translucent. Add the seared spare ribs back into the oven. Add rest of the ingredients for braising. Bring to the boil. Cover the lid of the Dutch oven. Close the dome of the grill.

7. Cook for 3- 3 ½ hours. Turn the ribs after 1-½ hours of cooking. Cook until tender. Remove the spareribs and set aside. When cool enough to handle, cut the spareribs.

8. Simmer the liquid in the Dutch oven uncovered until thick.

9. Pour sauce over the spareribs. Serve over roast potatoes or rice.

Stew Skewer

Ingredients:

- 8 cups vegetable broth
- 8 medium potatoes, peeled, cut into 1 cm thick slices
- 2 red onions, quartered
- Sea salt to taste
- 4 carrots, cut into 1 cm thick slices
- 2 smoked sausages, cut into 1 cm thick slices
- 18 bay leaves
- 7 tablespoons butter (optional)

Method:

1. Operate the grill following the instructions of the manufacturer. Set the Kamado grill for direct cooking. Set the temperature at 220 ° F.
2. Place a drip pan on the grid.
3. Add 4-6 apple or peach wood chunks in it.
4. Clean and grease the grill grates.
5. Meanwhile, place a saucepan with broth over medium heat. Add carrot and potato slices. Cook for 8 minutes. Drain and retain the broth in the saucepan. Let the broth simmer.
6. Place the carrots and potatoes in a bowl of cold water for a couple of minutes. Drain and set aside.
7. Thread the potatoes, carrots, onions, and sausages onto flat skewers. Insert bay leaves in each skewer in between. You will need 8 flat skewers.
8. Place the skewers on the drip pan with its ends on the edges of the drip pan.
9. Close the dome of the grill. Pour simmering broth in the drip pan. Cook for 25-30 minutes until tender.
10. Remove the skewers from the grill and remove the vegetables from the skewers and add to a bowl. Mash the vegetables and add the meat from the skewer.
11. Drizzle butter if using on it and serve.

Braised Carrots

Ingredients:

- 4 yellow carrots, trim the ends
- 4 orange carrots, trim the ends
- 4 purple carrots, trim the ends
- 2 sprigs licorice
- 2 red onions, cut into rings
- 2 sprigs thyme
- 4-5 tablespoons pumpkin seed oil
- 1 ½ large mandarins or Clementine's
- Pepper to taste
- Salt to taste
- 3 bay leaves
- 4-5 tablespoons apple cider or sherry vinegar
- Olive oil, as required

Method:

1. Operate the grill following the instructions of the manufacturer. Set the Kamado grill for direct cooking. Set the temperature at 175 ° F.
2. Add 4-6 apple or peach wood chunks in it. Place a grid.
3. Place a large sheet of wax paper on your work area. Place all the carrots, onion rings, bay leaves, thyme and licorice over it.
4. Pour pumpkin seed oil and vinegar over the vegetables. Juice the mandarins and pour over the carrot. Also, add the peels.
5. Cover with another sheet of wax paper. Fold only the edges of both the sheets of wax paper together a few times.
6. Place the wax paper packet on the grid. Close the dome of the grill. Cook for about an hour or until the carrots are tender. Shake the packet every 20 minutes while cooking.
7. Open the packets. The carrots may be golden brown in color. Serve with the cooked juices. Sprinkle salt, pepper, and some olive oil over it and serve.

Cake and Berry Cobbler

Ingredients:

- 3 cans (21 ounces each) raspberry pie filling
- 2 cups water
- 1 ½ packages yellow cake mix
- ¾ cup canola oil
- Vanilla ice cream to serve

Method:

1. Operate the grill following the instructions of the manufacturer. Set the Kamado grill for direct cooking. Set the temperature at 250° F.
2. Add 4-6 apple or peach wood chunks in it.
3. Take a cast iron Dutch oven and line it with heavy-duty aluminum foil. Pour apple pie filling into it.
4. Mix together in a bowl, cake mix, oil, and water. Pour over the pie filling. Place the Dutch oven directly on the charcoal. Cover the Dutch oven.
5. Cover the dome of the grill. Cook for about 40-45 minutes.
6. Serve warm with ice cream.

Pots of S'mores

Ingredients:

- 7.5 ounces whole graham crackers, crushed
- 7 ounces sweetened condensed milk
- ½ cup butterscotch chips
- ¼ cup butter, melted
- 1 cup semi sweet chocolate chips
- 1 cup miniature marshmallows

Method:

1. Operate the grill following the instructions of the manufacturer. Set the Kamado grill for direct cooking. Set the temperature at 250° F.
2. Add 4-6 apple or peach wood chunks in it.
3. Take a cast iron Dutch oven and line it with heavy-duty aluminum foil.
4. Add crackers and butter into the Dutch oven and mix well. Press it onto the bottom of the Dutch oven.
5. Pour milk. Sprinkle chocolate chips and butterscotch chips. Finally, sprinkle marshmallow. Place the Dutch oven on the grill.
6. Cover the Dutch oven and close the dome of the grill. Bake for 15 minutes or until set.
7. Serve warm.

Chapter 10: Kamado Grill Baking Recipes

Camp site Grilled Salmon

Ingredients:

- 2 pounds salmon fillets or steaks, about 1 inch thick, rinsed, pat dried
- 4 tablespoons dry sherry
- 2 tablespoons fresh ginger root, minced
- 2 scallions or green onions, thinly sliced
- 4 tablespoons soy sauce
- 2 tablespoon brown sugar
- 4 cloves garlic, minced

Method:

1. Add all the ingredients except green onions into a zip lock bag. Shake the bag to coat well. Chill for an hour
2. Operate the grill following the instructions of the manufacturer. Set the Kamado grill for baking with the temperature at 275-350 ° F for about 25-30 minutes.
3. Place lava stone or pizza stone on the grilling grate. Grease the pizza stone.
4. Place 3-6 mesquite or hickory wood chunks or wood chunks of your choice or 3-5 handfuls chips over the charcoal for smoking. Close the dome until you place the salmon.
5. Place the fish with its skin side down on the lava stone. Close the dome. Bake for around 10 minutes or until the fish flakes readily when pierced with a fork.

Chicken Croquettes

Ingredients:

- 4 tablespoons butter
- 4 teaspoons ground mustard
- ¼ teaspoon pepper powder or to taste
- 4 cups cooked chicken, chopped into small pieces or minced
- 2 tablespoons fresh parsley, minced
- 2 teaspoons lemon juice
- ¼ teaspoon cayenne pepper or to taste
- 2 eggs
- 6 tablespoons all-purpose flour
- ½ teaspoon salt or to taste
- 2 cups milk
- ½ cup green bell pepper, chopped
- 1 small onion, minced
- ½ teaspoon paprika
- 3 cups bread crumbs
- 2-3 tablespoons water

Method:

1. Place a saucepan over medium heat. Add butter. When butter melts, add flour, mustard, salt, and pepper and sauté for about a minute,
2. Add milk, stirring constantly. Keep stirring until the mixture becomes thick. Turn off the heat.
3. Add chicken, parsley, paprika, cayenne, bell pepper and lemon juice. Mix well. Taste and adjust the seasonings if necessary.
4. Place the mixture in the refrigerator for 3-4 hours.
5. Operate the grill following the instructions of the manufacturer. Set the Kamado grill for baking with the temperature at 375 ° F for about 25-30 minutes.
6. Remove the mixture from the refrigerator about 30 minutes before grilling. Divide the mixture into 8-10 equal portions. Shape into croquettes.

7. Add breadcrumbs into a shallow bowl. Add eggs and water into another bowl. Beat lightly.
8. Grease a baking sheet with cooking spray. Set aside.
9. First, dredge the croquettes in bread crumbs. Next dip in egg mixture and again in breadcrumbs. Place on the prepared baking sheet.
10. Place the baking sheet near the top of the dome of the Kamado grill. Cook for about 20 minutes or until done. Turn the croquettes after 10-12 minutes of cooking.

Classic Margherita Pizza

Ingredients:

- A ball of pizza dough of about 10-12 ounces, risen to room temperature
- 4 teaspoons extra virgin olive oil
- 2 sprigs parsley, chopped
- 1 teaspoon dried oregano
- Freshly ground pepper to taste
- Salt to taste
- A handful fresh basil leaves, chopped
- 1 medium onion, sliced
- 3 teaspoons garlic, minced
- 2 ½ cups canned, whole, peeled tomatoes
- 5 ounces fresh mozzarella, thinly sliced

Method:

1. To make Margherita sauce: Place a skillet over medium heat. Add oil. When the oil is heated, add onions and parsley and sauté until golden brown.
2. Add garlic and oregano and sauté until fragrant. Add tomatoes and cook. Crush it simultaneously as it cooks.
3. Simmer until the sauce thickens. Remove from heat and set aside.
4. Operate the grill following the instructions of the manufacturer. Set the Kamado grill for baking with the temperature at 650 ° F for about 25-30 minutes.
5. Place a pizza stone at the point of opening of the grill.
6. To assemble the pizza: Place the pizza dough on a pizza peel that is sprinkled with cornmeal.
7. Spread some of the Margherita sauce over the pizza dough.
8. Place the slices of mozzarella all over the sauce.
9. Carefully slide the pizza onto the pizza stone. Bake for 18-20 minutes. Sprinkle the basil leaves after 15 minutes of baking.
10. When done, slice into wedges and serve.

Zucchini Bread

Ingredients:

- 4 ½ cups zucchini, shredded
- 1 cup vegetable oil
- 6 eggs
- ¾ cup walnuts or pecans
- 1 ½ teaspoons salt
- ¾ teaspoon ground cloves
- 2 ½ cups sugar
- 3 teaspoons vanilla extract
- 4 ½ cups all purpose flour
- 6 teaspoons baking powder
- 1 ½ teaspoons ground cinnamon

Method:

1. Operate the grill following the instructions of the manufacturer. Set the Kamado grill for indirect cooking with the temperature at 350 ° F for about 25-30 minutes.
2. Place the heat deflector with the ceramic plate in bottom position in the grill. Place the grill grate on top.
3. Add 4-6 apple or peach wood chunks in it.
4. Mix together all the ingredients in a bowl. Transfer the dough into either 2 greased loaf pans or 1 large loaf pan.
5. Place the loaf pans or pan on the grill. Bake for 45-60 minutes or until done.
6. When done, remove from the grill. Cool for a while. Remove from the loaf pan.
7. Slice and serve.

Open Faced Spaghetti Pot Pie

Ingredients:

- 2 slices provolone
- 2 cups cooked angel hair pasta
- ½ cup ricotta cheese
- 2 eggs
- Salt to taste
- Pepper to taste
- 1 bulb burrata cheese
- 1 ½ cups tomato sauce (you can use store bought one or refer Margherita pizza recipe for the sauce)
- 1 cup Romano parmesan cheese, grated
- A handful fresh basil, chopped
- 1-pound pizza dough

Method:

1. Operate the grill following the instructions of the manufacturer. Set the Kamado grill for indirect cooking with the temperature at 350 ° F for about 25-30 minutes.
2. Place the heat deflector with the ceramic plate in bottom position in the grill. Place the grill grate on top.
3. Add 4-6 apple or peach wood chunks in it.
4. Take 2 ramekins and grease with cooking spray.
5. Place a slice of provolone at the bottom of each of the ramekins.
6. Add half bulb burrata cheese in each. Top the burrata cheese with a cup of angel hair pasta.
7. Divide and spoon the tomato sauce over it.
8. Divide and place ricotta cheese over the tomato sauce.
9. Sprinkle salt, pepper and Parmesan cheese.
10. Divide the dough into 2 equal portions. Roll each portion of the dough into rounds as you do in a pizza. It should be rolled at least an inch bigger than the diameter of the ramekin.

11. Place each of the rolled dough on each of the ramekins. It should cover the ingredients of the ramekins completely and also hang up to half the length of the ramekin.
12. Brush the dough with beaten egg. Take a sharp knife and make cuts on the dough in a few places.
13. Now place the ramekins on the grill. The dough should face the top.
14. Bake for 20-25 minutes.
15. When done, remove the ramekins and cool for 5-6 minutes. Place on the plate. Carefully remove the pot pie with the help of a fork by loosening the edges.
16. Sprinkle some more cheese and basil. Spoon some more sauce if desired and serve.

Jalapeño Cheddar Skillet Cornbread

Ingredients:

For the dry ingredients:

- 2 ½ cups cornmeal
- ½ cup sugar
- 1 teaspoon baking soda
- 1 ½ cups all purpose flour
- 1 teaspoon kosher salt
- 4 teaspoons baking powder

For the wet ingredients:

- 4 eggs
- ½ cup sour cream
- 2 cups sharp cheddar cheese, shredded, divided
- 10 tablespoons butter, unsalted
- 2 cups buttermilk
- 8 tablespoons pickled diced jalapeños
- ½ cup milk

Method:

1. Operate the grill following the instructions of the manufacturer. Set the Kamado grill for indirect cooking with the temperature at 350 ° F for about 25-30 minutes.
2. Place the heat deflector with the ceramic plate in bottom position in the grill. Place the grill grate on top.
3. Add 4-6 apple or peach wood chunks in it.
4. Place a cast iron skillet on the grill grate. Add some butter. When butter melts, remove the skillet from the grill. Swirl the pan so that the butter spreads all over the bottom as well as the sides of the pan. Set aside.
5. Add all the dry ingredients into a large bowl. Whisk until well combined.
6. Add all the wet ingredients (retain ½ the cheese) into the bowl of dry ingredients. Also, pour the melted butter and whisk until well combined.

7. Pour the batter into the cast iron skillet that should be warm by now.
8. Swirl the skillet once more so that the batter spreads evenly. Sprinkle the retained cheese all over it.
9. Place the skillet on the grill. Bake for 45-60 minutes or until done.
10. When done, remove from the grill. Cool for a while.
11. Slice and serve.

Chicken Alfredo Pizza

Ingredients:

- 1 refrigerated pizza dough
- ½ pound grilled chicken strips, boneless
- A handful spinach leaves, chopped
- ½ jar Ragu Alfredo sauce with mushrooms
- ½ pound mozzarella cheese, shredded

Method:

1. Operate the grill following the instructions of the manufacturer. Set the Kamado grill for baking with the temperature at 450 ° F for about 25-30 minutes.
2. Place a pizza stone at the point of opening of the grill.
3. To assemble the pizza: Place the pizza dough on a pizza peel, which is sprinkled with cornmeal.
4. Spread Alfredo sauce over the pizza dough.
5. Place the chicken strips on the dough. Sprinkle spinach leaves over it. Sprinkle mozzarella all over the pizza.
6. Carefully slide the pizza onto the pizza stone. Bake for 12--15 minutes.
7. When done, slice into wedges and serve.

Blueberry French Toast Casserole

Ingredients:

- 7-8 slices white bread, chopped
- 1 cup half and half
- 4 large eggs
- ½ cup milk
- ½ tablespoon vanilla extract
- ¼ cup butter, salted, melted, cooled
- Maple syrup, warmed, to serve
- ½ pound breakfast sausage, crumbled after cooking
- 1 tablespoon firmly packed light brown sugar
- ¼ teaspoon kosher salt
- 2 ounces fresh blueberries

Method:

1. Add bread and sausage into a bowl and mix well.
2. Add eggs into another bowl and whisk well. Add butter and whisk until well combined. Pour over the bread. Mix well. Press the bread down.
3. Transfer into a greased baking dish. Sprinkle blueberries on it. Press the blueberries down slightly into the bread. Cover with cling wrap or foil.
4. Refrigerate for 6-8 hours. Remove from the refrigerator an hour before baking
5. Operate the grill following the instructions of the manufacturer. Set the Kamado grill for baking with the temperature at 350 ° F for about 25-30 minutes. Set for indirect cooking.
6. Place the heat deflector with the ceramic plate on the grill.
7. Add 4-6 apple or peach wood chunks in it.
8. Remove the foil. Place the baking dish on the grid. Bake for 40-50minutes or until firm in the center. Rotate the dish by 180 ° half way through baking.
9. Remove from the grill and cool for a while.
10. Serve warm with a drizzle of maple syrup.

Garlic Toast

Ingredients:

- ½ loaf French bread, cut into 1-inch thick slices
- Salt to taste
- ¼ cup garlic infused olive oil

Method:

1. Operate the grill following the instructions of the manufacturer. Set the Kamado grill for baking with the temperature at 325 ° F for about 25-30 minutes. Set for indirect cooking.
2. Place the heat deflector with the ceramic plate on the grill.
3. Add 4-6 apple or peach wood chunks in it.
4. Brush bread slices with oil. Sprinkle salt and place on the grill.
5. Bake for 5 minutes or until toasted.

Dump Cake

Ingredients:

- 30 ounces canned cherry pie filling
- 30 ounces canned crushed pineapple
- 1 ½ boxes yellow cake mix
- 3 sticks butter
- 1 ½ bags pecan pieces

Method:

1. Operate the grill following the instructions of the manufacturer. Set the Kamado grill for baking with the temperature at 350 ° F for about 25-30 minutes. Set for indirect cooking.
2. Add wood chunks in it.
3. Place the heat deflector with the ceramic plate on the grill.
4. Add all the ingredients into a bowl. Mix well. Pour into a Dutch oven or baking accessory. Place on the grill. Cover the dome.
5. Bake for 45 -60 minutes. Remove from the grill. Cool for a while. Slice and serve warm or cold.

Cranberry Pear Crumble

Ingredients:

- 6 medium ripe pears, peeled, cored, sliced
- ½ cup sugar
- ½ teaspoon ground cinnamon
- 1 cup dried cranberries
- 4 tablespoons all-purpose flour
- 2 tablespoons butter

For the topping:

- 4 tablespoons butter, melted
- 2 cups granola without raisins
- ½ teaspoon ground cinnamon

Method:

1. Add pear slices and cranberries into a bowl. Sprinkle sugar, flour, and cinnamon over it. Toss well.
2. Operate the grill following the instructions of the manufacturer. Set the Kamado grill for baking with the temperature at 350 ° F for about 25-30 minutes. Set for indirect cooking.
3. Add wood chunks in it.
4. Place the heat deflector with the ceramic plate on the grill.
5. Place a cast iron skillet over the grill. Add butter. When butter melts, add pear mixture and mix well. Cover the dome of the grill. Bake for 30-40 minutes. Stir once half way through baking.

Chapter 11: Kamado Conversion Chart

Beef, veal chops, lambs

Roasts & Steaks

Smoking   125 F

Roasting/baking   125 F

Grilling   135 F

Searing   145-155 F

Pork

Pork chops

Smoking   125 F

Roasting/baking   130 F

Grilling   140 F

Searing   155-160 F

Pork Ham (Fresh)

For smoking, roasting or baking - Use roasting or smoking temperature guide

Searing   135-140 F

Shoulder

For smoking, roasting or baking - Use roasting or smoking temperature guide

Searing   200 F

Poultry (Whole & Pieces)

For smoking, roasting or baking - Use roasting or smoking temperature guide

Searing   160-165 F

Seafood

Finfish

For smoking, roasting or baking- Cook until it turns opaque and can be easily separated using a fork

Searing   145 F

Crab, Lobster & Shrimp

For smoking, roasting, searing or baking - Cook until the flesh turns translucent

Clams and oysters

For smoking, roasting, searing or baking - Cook until the shell automatically open during cooking

Scallops

For smoking, roasting, searing or baking - Cook until the flesh is translucent, milky white and firm

Conclusion

I hope you enjoyed reading every bit of this book because I have had some great fun writing it. I have been using the Kamado grill and smoker for about a year now, and I am pleasantly satisfied with the results.

If you haven't bought the Kamado smoker and grill yet, it's about time you should consider buying one. Investing in a device like the Kamado will not only make your food tastier, but it will also cut down on your expenses. There's so much information floating around the market about the Kamado that it can be overwhelming for a prospective buyer. We understood this and wanted to ensure that our readers know everything about this device beforehand.

I sincerely hope that this guide was successful in clarifying all your doubts about the Kamado grill and smoker. Don't forget to write me and let me know how you liked the book. I will be looking forward to your responses.

CPSIA information can be obtained
at www.ICGtesting.com
Printed in the USA
BVHW052049130820
586209BV00012B/61

9 781952 117046